HIDDEN DANGERS IN WHAT
WE EAT AND DRINK

Jan de Vries

Healthcare series

HIDDEN DANGERS IN WHAT WE EAT AND DRINK

A Lifelong Guide to Healthy Living

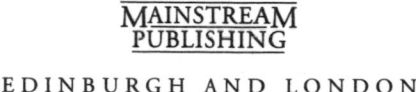

MAINSTREAM
PUBLISHING

EDINBURGH AND LONDON

First published in Great Britain in 2003 by
MAINSTREAM PUBLISHING (EDINBURGH) LTD
7 Albany Street
Edinburgh EH1 3UG

ISBN 1 84018 516 3

A catalogue record for this book is available from the British Library

Typeset in Baskerville MT and Garamond

Printed in Great Britain by
Cox & Wyman Ltd

CONTENTS

Preface   7
Chapter 1:   A Perfectly Normal Child   15
Chapter 2:   How to Make a Healthy Baby   18
Chapter 3:   Pregnancy and Childbirth   24
Chapter 4:   Breast-feeding your Baby   29
Chapter 5:   Breast-feeding and Wet-nurses   38
Chapter 6:   How to Feed your Baby or Toddler   43
Chapter 7:   Aggressive Toddlers   46
Chapter 8:   Children with Learning Disabilities   50
Chapter 9:   Different Symptoms   53
Chapter 10: Possible Causes   58
Chapter 11: What's Wrong with our Food?   62
Chapter 12: Soft Drinks – Beware!   67
Chapter 13: Sugar   71
Chapter 14: Low Blood Sugar   75
Chapter 15: Food Allergies and Incompatibilities   80
Chapter 16: The Phosphorus Connection   86
Chapter 17: Food Additives   89
Chapter 18: Indirect Food Additives   94
Chapter 19: Dangerous Metals   96
Chapter 20: Salicylates   102
Chapter 21: A Lack of Nutrients   106
Chapter 22: Noise   108
Chapter 23: E Numbers and Other Dangers   112
Chapter 24: Modern Medicine   118

Chapter 25: Ritalin and Other Strong Drugs 122
Chapter 26: Child Psychiatry 126
Chapter 27: Homoeopathy 131
Chapter 28: Helping with Herbs 138
Chapter 29: Orthomolecular Medicine 141
Chapter 30: The Importance of Light 145
Chapter 31: Food and Criminal Behaviour 149
Chapter 32: Cleansing the Organism, Detoxifying the Body 155
Chapter 33: Stress, Addiction and Drugs 158
Index 174

PREFACE

Writing this book, I hope to make my readers aware of an alarming and extremely dangerous development that began about a century ago as a consequence of our so-called progress. Our wonderful new world has lost much of its original beauty and now seems to be full of menace, of which, up to now, we have barely been aware. Although our children are most affected by these environmental dangers, our own physical and mental health is also gradually being destroyed as a consequence of increasing pollution. It is not only our environment that is being polluted, but also the inside of our body: our organs, tissues, blood and cells, nervous system and brain are being polluted slowly but surely, day by day. We are still ignorant about this and do not realise that the first signs of a general degeneration and collapse are to be seen all over; the behavioural changes in our children are only the tip of the iceberg.

Many people, including some of those who govern us, suffer from so much internal pollution, that normal thought and behaviour is out of the question.

There is an old saying, 'A healthy mind in a healthy body' – when the organism of a person is filled with waste products, their mind cannot be healthy. The pollution of our inner and outer environments is at the root of many wrong decisions and political disasters. It influences our life on all levels, and may be one of the main causes of the imminent destruction of our world.

Our children are the innocent victims of this general malaise. Many problems have grown out of all proportion and taken on epidemic dimensions. We know that something is very wrong with modern society, but the phenomenon is like the many-headed Hydra, or an octopus whose tentacles are interwoven with almost every aspect of modern society. Even those who realise the danger do not know how to unravel the threads of the net in which we, to a greater or lesser extent, have been caught. If we continue in this way it means a slow and terrible death and the end of civilisation. Many of us have given up hope, but some of us still want to try and save some of the old values before it is too late. The first thing we must do is save our children.

More and more children in our affluent society are ill, not only physically but also to a certain degree mentally and emotionally. They are the innocent bystanders and victims of the lassitude of our generation, and of former generations. When selfish, greedy and ignorant people poisoned and changed our living soil into an infertile substance we did not protest. Under the pretence of helping humanity in its fight against hunger they maltreated healthy, natural food in every way possible, adding innumerable chemical substances. They took away all that was valuable and turned it into lifeless, artificial products that do not deserve to be called food. Even people in the so-called underdeveloped countries would become ill if this kind of food was their daily fare. Most of the colours, smells and tastes of such products are factory-made, but who cares? Supermarket carts are loaded with these artificial foods and drinks, and because they are colourful and taste good our children love them.

Few people seem to realise that poor-quality soil treated with chemical fertilisers and artificial 'food' filled with additives can only support us at a low level of health. Many valuable nutrients have been destroyed and chemical substances that are extremely toxic, especially for sensitive young children, have taken their place.

Our brain is the most vulnerable part of our body and we know that one-third of all the nutrients we ingest are used by the brain. No wonder that millions of children (and many adults) in our western countries are suffering from nervousness, sleeplessness, hyperactivity and, even worse, mental problems, which are increasing at a frightening rate. Hundreds of millions of tranquillisers are being prescribed and children who take these often act like zombies. When they grow up, many of these children never become responsible citizens and often land in jail or in mental institutions.

This is hardly ever the fault of desperate parents or teachers, who themselves feel helpless and insecure. Nothing will help as long as these parents are not able to find the right physician, who can get to the heart of the matter. Such a physician will forbid all junk food, soft drinks, sweets and any kind of refined food, and take other natural, much needed measures.

Those who have never been confronted with these problems have no idea of the terrible stress parents of hyperactive and mentally disturbed children have to endure. The children themselves are not to blame, as they cannot control their behaviour. They are the victims of compulsive obsessions and most of them suffer even more than their parents do. These problems are due to bad functioning of a part of their little brain, which most often has been caused by a lack of some specific nutrients and/or of a surplus of certain toxic substances.

As the metabolism of every child functions differently and individually, and as each child reacts in its own way to certain substances, it is very difficult and sometimes almost impossible to find out which toxins are responsible. However, we know about some basic dangers that threaten our children and we also know that behavioural problems are never due to only one single cause, but always to a combination of many different negative influences.

Of course, there are some cases of brain injuries or real diseases of the brain and the nervous system, however, children suffering from these make up only a very small percentage when compared to other children with behavioural problems. In this book I will concentrate only on children who come into the last category and this is by far the largest group.

Behavioural problems have become a very big problem and will be a major worry for us in the near future. A few decades ago the first tell-tale signs of this calamity became visible. In almost every school class there are children with such problems and teaching often becomes a nearly impossible task. There is an increasing nervousness, as well as yelling and screaming and the loss of respect for the elder generation. When kids are only 11 or 12 years old, many of them start smoking and drinking. Later there are also drug abuse, burglary and knife fights and as these problems accelerate there are suicide, rape, murder and other criminal behaviour. Other young people are diagnosed schizophrenic or mentally unbalanced and land, sometimes for life, in jail or in different institutions.

On the Internet I found a very interesting summary about the changes that have taken place since 1940, concerning the behaviour of schoolchildren.

THE GOOD OLD DAYS

1940	*Today*
Talking	drug abuse
chewing gum	alcohol abuse
making noise	pregnancy
running in the hallways	suicide
getting out of place in line	rape
wearing improper clothing	robbery
not putting paper in the wastebasket	assault/burglary
	criminal
	behaviour

This overview is related to problems in the United States. However, we will not have to wait long before we see the same things happen in Europe.

And that is only part of the story. The changes we see in our youth have taken place in all layers of our society. We do not trust each other any more. Honesty is going down the drain. Business is mainly based on knowing how to take advantage of other people and make as much money as possible – in what manner is less important. Politicians sell their own countries for money and bankers only work for big profits. Helping others is seen as worthwhile only if there is a profit to be made and any difference of opinion, for example in religion, is an excellent excuse for fighting and starting a war.

Of course the older generation were never angels, but things have altered so drastically in the last 50 to 100 years that nobody feels safe any more. Why did this change happen, and what is the cause of it? People cannot have changed so much in so short a time. Parents still love their children, and children love their parents. Most teachers have chosen their profession because they like children and want to help them. People still dream their dreams, but many of those dreams have become nightmares.

What has changed in our lives and those of our children to make such behaviour possible? What kind of change has happened? There is only one possible answer to these questions. There is nothing that has changed as profoundly and completely over the last few decades as our eating habits.

'Junk food' was an American invention, as were soft drinks. The main dangers to our health in these foods are refined sugar, refined flour, refined oils and, above all, thousands and thousands of chemical additives. Almost everything we eat and drink nowadays has been changed from a natural into an unnatural product, and processed and infiltrated with uncountable chemicals.

Young children are very sensitive, more sensitive than grown-ups, and their immune system and digestive organs are even less able than ours to assimilate all the different foreign substances incorporated into our food.

As many of these chemicals cannot be neutralised or excreted from the body right away, they circulate in our body fluids and reach all our body cells, including those of our brain.

The inner defensive mechanisms of young children react very strongly to toxins and poisons. Even the smallest quantity of a toxic substance, for example from a small sweet or a salty cracker, may provoke immediate allergic reactions in a child. These reactions may include hyperactivity, or any other kind of personality change. We should not blame our government for all the toxins that are in circulation, as much research has been done in this area. All new substances are thoroughly checked before being pronounced 'safe' and given an 'E number'. But even for governments it is an impossible task to keep track of the hundreds of new chemical substances that are being presented each year. Many tests on healthy animals, using cell cultures or other means, are done with the intention of finding out in what way toxins can harm the human body and cause diseases. But tests on humans, to find out the effects on the mind and behaviour, when hundreds of extremely small quantities of toxins accumulate and combine to increase their potential toxicity, have never been done. Therefore, no government can be sure how many of these substances really are harmless for the unborn child or sensitive children.

Safety margins are indicated for the specific quantity of additives allowed, in order to prevent physical disease. However, it is a fact that many children eat large quantities of foods they like. In this way they ingest far more of a certain additive than is considered 'safe'. Some children are more sensitive than others, and no one knows yet what dangers the interactions of the many different chemicals in our daily food present; we see only the tragic results. In Chapter 23 I will give you a list of the E numbers it would be best to avoid. Colour- and taste-enhancing additives especially can be extremely dangerous, and seem to be one of the main causes of hyperactivity and other personality changes in children. Children love nice colours and those who market sweets are very much aware of this. Even if your children are in good health and you permit them to have a sweet once in a while, watch out for food colourings. Some may be really harmless but others might, in a short or a longer time, change your sweet and obedient child into a little monster.

It is not only food colourings and sweets that can be harmful to your children. Milk and milk products, some cereals, peanut butter and other refined and natural foods may in part be responsible for personality changes or even problems that are far more serious. This is only the tip of the iceberg – the real effects of such problems await us in the near future.

There have been many other changes in the environment, but food is the most direct and intimate contact we all have with our environment. Strong toxic substances are used, for example, in agriculture and almost everything we eat has been treated and altered in some way or other. Many medical drugs are also toxic or contain toxic ingredients that provoke allergies and other, more dangerous side-effects. Toxic chemicals are part of our civilisation.

They have been used for the production of most commodities in modern life. These chemicals are fine when they help us to make things easier and give us the opportunity to enjoy life more. Chemical substances should be able to help us, but they should not be used as a means to improve the external appearance of sweets, desserts and other foodstuffs that children like to eat.

Personality changes in children resulting from chemical additives have been observed by many conscientious scientists and physicians for a long time already. The saddest thing is that such children may stay hyperactive, depressed or suffer from an even worse fate for the rest of their lives. The one thing parents can do right away when such problems appear is to watch the eating habits of their children and find out which are the worst culprits.

In the following chapters I will explain the effects of the hidden dangers in our diet and environment on our health, even before birth. Step by step I will take you on a journey, starting at the very beginning of life, in order to reveal the full extent of the damage that may be done, and how we can help improve our own and our children's well-being. After reading this book you will agree that we have to do something; we must intervene before it is too late.

❧ Chapter 1 ❧

A PERFECTLY NORMAL CHILD

Some children are very quiet and some are extremely active. We should always remember that most children have more energy at their disposal than we do, and they have to somehow get this surplus of energy out of their system. Some small children like to look at picture books, while others prefer to run around for hours. That depends on the character of the child, on its hereditary disposition, on momentary emotions, on the weather and on hundreds of other things. Once in a while every child behaves in an unexpected way, and that is completely normal. If a child is bad, he or she usually regrets their behaviour after a while. It is completely normal for a child to be sad or in a bad mood sometimes. Grown-up people sometimes act in the same way. We are all human and everyone has shortcomings and needs to let off steam occasionally.

Never make the mistake of labelling a child that is either extremely active or very quiet as 'hyperactive' or 'autistic' before you and your physician are completely sure of the diagnosis. Some children often exhibit exaggerated but perfectly normal development. Not every child who is overly active, inattentive or impulsive has a behavioural disorder. You can ruin the lives of children forever by making them out to be different from their friends. First find out if there are any deep-seated emotional or personal problems bothering your child, and then help them sort things out and become happy again. Children live much more intensively than we do, and they take real or imagined problems much more to heart. However, when a child's bad behaviour, aggression, hostility or stress becomes permanent, something may be very wrong indeed.

Such children are certainly not happy. Although many of them are very intelligent, they cannot concentrate and are easily distracted. For most of them it is impossible to keep quiet and sit still for more than a few minutes. Others react in exactly the opposite way and hardly ever show any reaction at all; they are 'autistic'.

All these children suffer from behavioural disorders that are still a puzzle for psychologists or psychiatrists, as well as for regular physicians. As yet nobody seems to know what is really the matter with these children and why their behaviour can be so strange. These abnormal behaviour patterns have been given many different names. Physicians once thought that they were symptoms of a brain disease and labelled the condition 'minimal brain damage' or 'minimal brain dysfunction' (MBD). Later on, this condition was called 'Attention Deficit Disorder' (ADD) or 'Attention Deficit Hyperactive Disorder' (AD/HD). The opposite kind of behaviour disorder, 'autism', is even more frightening. Children suffering from autism seem to be wrapped up in a cocoon and show hardly any reactions at all.

Both kinds of behaviour disorders, hyperactivity and autism, are increasing with frightening speed. In our western world there are millions of children suffering from them. One estimate in the United States quotes 2.4 million, and another quotes 4 million with AD/HD. Most of these children have learning and/or reading disabilities. In Europe the numbers seem to be a little lower, but they are fast catching up. Over 7 million children in the USA take mind-altering, psychotropic drugs with dangerous side-effects and the sale of Ritalin, the most frequently prescribed drug, has increased as much as 400 per cent in five years.

Unfortunately, all these medications are potentially harmful and only mask the symptoms without getting to the core of the problem. The potential risks of such drugs are a high price to pay to ease parents' worries and make teachers' jobs easier; they often turn a child into something resembling a vegetable.

There are many different causes of behavioural deficiencies and in order to help such children, their entire lifestyle and eating habits, as well as those of their family, should be studied in order to find out when and under what circumstances the strange behaviour started. Each child is an individual human being and when setting up a treatment programme many things have to be taken into consideration.

Even before your baby is born, while you are pregnant and also while your baby is still small, you can try to prevent your child becoming hyperactive or autistic. If you want to have healthy and happy children, there is much you can do yourself in order to fulfil your wish.

Chapter 2

HOW TO MAKE A HEALTHY BABY

In order to cultivate healthy plants a farmer needs to have healthy seeds, and seeds can only be healthy when they come from healthy plants, growing in a healthy soil, containing all the different nutrients plants need. Everything in nature functions according to the same basic laws, and the creation of a human being is no exception to the rule.

At the time of conception human 'seeds' must also be healthy. Both husband and wife are responsible for the health and well-being of their future child and must therefore, even before the child is conceived, pay attention to their food selection and living habits. They do not need to be fanatics or health-nuts, but they should make it a habit to eat simple, wholesome meals, get more sleep and exercise and, above all, avoid the use of potentially gene-altering substances such as recreational drugs, alcohol and nicotine.

The original word 'honeymoon' comes from northern Europe and means 'going into hiding'. However, in many European languages the word 'honeymoon' has a connection with the words 'honey' and 'moon' and the origin of these words lies in the use of old customs. However, the German term for honeymoon is '*hochzeit*', derived from two words, '*höchste*' and '*zeit*', which in English means 'high time'. Long engagements were, until about 100 years ago, needed, because the bride could not be married until her dowry was complete. As the preparation of the dowry often took a long time, it could happen that there was already a child on the way and it was 'high time' that the marriage took place.

Going away together after marriage is a very old custom. In the Middle Ages, when a man wanted a child, he often abducted a woman and went into hiding with her during a phase of the moon (for about a month). During this time it was the custom that every day both of them should drink some honeyed wine (mead), which was said to improve fertility. The custom of abducting the bride and drinking mead is an ancient one.

Honeyed wine (mead) was made from a mixture of honey, water and fruit juices undergoing a fermentation process and it is thought that this was the first alcoholic drink people produced.

We know now that honey contains many different vitamins, minerals, enzymes, hormones and other important substances and therefore it seems to be quite possible that honey increases fertility. At the same time a reluctant bride, under the influence of the light alcohol content of honeyed wine, became more pliable. For the same reason, a little wine during the honeymoon will help newlyweds to relax together. However, although a little wine does not hurt, hard alcoholic drinks should definitely not be touched while honeymooning.

After their marriage most people go on a honeymoon in order to relax, to get to know one another more intimately, to have a lovely holiday and to be happy.

The most important objective, however, is to get away from other people and, if possible, to start creating their first child. When planning a honeymoon, some people go on a cruise, while others prefer to go to a nice hotel in some big city they have always wanted to visit. Both choices are wrong if the couple plans to start a family. The original idea of a honeymoon is to get away from people and to relax. Big cities and cruises may be fine for a normal holiday, but at the start of married life, they are the wrong choice. On cruises and in big cities relaxation is not possible.

Many people today still have ritualistic celebrations in homage to the gods of fertility. In olden times the only chance of survival was often to have many children, and so the fertility of human beings and domestic animals has always been very important.

Nature is very wise. When people are not healthy, it will be very difficult or even impossible for them to have a baby. Causes of infertility include a wide range of physical, emotional and environmental factors. The 'seeds' of some men are too weak or the sperm count is too low. Some women will not be able to accept the sperm of the man because of ovulation dysfunction. This can be due to poor nutrition, hormonal imbalance, ovarian cysts, an abnormal uterus, a past history of pelvic inflammatory diseases and other problems.

Not long ago, there was an article in the Austrian newspaper *Die Presse* which was headed: 'Sperm quality is going down continuously'. It said: 'Because of chemical pollution, according to university professor Dr Walter Ludvik, the sperm quality in men has decreased 30 per cent during the last three decades.' For this, the professor blames the destruction of the environment; exhaust fumes; heavy metals, for example lead; fertilisers; preservatives and pesticides. People take in all these toxins with their daily nutrition and when they use polluted water for drinking and cooking.

Newsweek reported that since 1938 the average sperm count had decreased by 50 per cent and at the same time the number of patients suffering from cancer of the prostate had trebled. In 1940 it was estimated that about 7 million American men suffered from 'erection dysfunction'. Now the estimates are between 15 and 25 million and when partial impotence is included this goes up to about 30 million. In Europe these estimates are also pretty high.

Sometimes it is very difficult for a physician to find out the actual reason for infertility, but often the problem is due to stress or an unhealthy lifestyle and can be remedied. Often, when both partners have changed their eating and living habits, in due course the woman will become pregnant. I have often seen this happen, even in the case of couples who had already given up all hope.

I still remember the day a Greek lady came to see me. She and her husband had been married for over six years. They were longing to have a child and both had seen several specialists. These physicians conducted many tests, but there seemed to be nothing really wrong and their reproductive organs were healthy. It was probably just a question of too much stress; they should try to relax more and enjoy life. If this brought no results, their last physician recommended that they should see a psychiatrist.

When she came to see me this Greek lady was quite desperate. She was not so young any more and soon it would be too late for her to have a child.

I spoke with her for a long time and enquired about their eating and living habits. It turned out that twice a week they went out to eat at a snack bar and at home they often ate ready meals. Both had a lack of fresh vegetables and never ate wholemeal bread, cereal or other such things.

The lady told me that when she and her husband were engaged they often used to go hiking or swimming, but that since their marriage they hardly did any exercise or sports any more and only seldom went for a walk. I advised her to take these good habits up again. Also, I recommended that from now on they should eat more home-made, fresh and wholesome food.

They both had a hair test done and when a week later the results of this test came back, it turned out that both of them had a lack of certain vitamins and minerals, which I prescribed in high doses. The lady suffered from toxic quantities of copper and mercury and therefore it was no wonder that she could not conceive. I prescribed a homoeopathic remedy that would help to eliminate these toxins from her body.

After two months the couple came to see me again. They were very happy and thanked me profusely, as the lady was now expecting her first child. The only problem for me was the fact that thereafter my office resembled a meeting place for Greek ladies who wanted to have children!

Modern food is lacking in many nutrients needed by our future citizens, and it would be good if young couples who were unable to procreate after a couple of years of trying had a hair test done in order to find out what vitamins or minerals are lacking. Hair tests are much more reliable than blood tests. This is due to the fact that the composition of the blood changes every so often. Hair taken from the neck of the person in question indicates any possible lack of nutrients. Also, any accumulation of toxins will be revealed. Some toxins, especially from certain heavy metals or medicines, can cause health problems that prevent conception. Our modern world is full of toxins and almost each day new and dangerous toxins are being used in industry or are added to our food.

Men have their own biochemical problems. Typically, men often are short of zinc. Zinc is the controlling element for male sexuality because it regulates testosterone levels. Testosterone levels dictate a man's (and a woman's) sexual appetite, his physical stamina and his sperm count. Low zinc levels also affect the sperm's mobility or ability to swim against the current. Normal zinc levels improve all of these. Old wives tales about oysters being a great aphrodisiac are scientifically correct. Oysters are loaded with zinc. They are great for men wanting to make babies. Other foods high in zinc are beef (*lean*), crab eggs, sunflower seeds, trout and wheat bran.

Deficiencies are often easy to fix because, if they are not too serious, one can simply eat more of the necessary foods and take the necessary supplements. Toxicity is a bigger problem; it may take a year to effectively deal with extreme toxicity. Toxins usually are lodged in every body cell. However, eating the right foods can naturally speed things up.

Sophia Loren longed for a baby. The beautiful movie star, with the world at her feet, could not get the one thing she wanted most: a cherished son or daughter. After dozens of tests and years of heartbreak, her doctors finally discovered she was toxic with copper. After the physicians corrected her copper imbalance, she conceived immediately.

If you have been unable to get pregnant and your doctor can't tell you why, since all your reproductive organs are in good health, the chances are that you, your partner, or both have a biochemical imbalance. You also should know that unless three distinct trace elements, copper, calcium and zinc, are stored in your body in the proper amounts, it is impossible for a woman to conceive or carry a baby to term or for a man to impregnate her.

Although our body needs a small amount of copper in order to stay healthy, copper imbalance often seems to be the major cause of unexplained infertility. We know that the brain controls fertility in both men and women, and in order to function correctly it needs some copper. However, too much has exactly the opposite effect. The copper/zinc ratio in your body regulates ovulation. If there is too much copper and too little zinc, a woman's fertility can be compromised. The imbalance can cause tumours and cysts to grow in the body, making it difficult to conceive. If a woman whose body contains too much copper does have a baby, there may be birth defects and the brain development of the baby may be adversely affected. Copper is not only found in water pipes and kitchenware, but also in birth control pills.

This is only one example of the complicated interaction of substances in our body. You will understand how important it is for your health to prevent the toxic influence from heavy metals. If you are interested in this, please see Chapter 19, 'Dangerous Metals'. Being aware of all these things is vital if you want to conceive a healthy and happy baby. However, the intuitive understanding of a loving mother once the baby is born can be even more important.

❧ Chapter 3 ❧

PREGNANCY AND CHILDBIRTH

Pregnancy is a very important episode in the life of a woman. Creating a baby is a work of art, and means serious and hard work. If you want to produce a perfect little baby you will have to work very hard at it, but human beings are creatures of habit and it is not always easy to give up the habits one has grown fond of. However, by simply improving your diet where improvement is necessary, you can greatly influence the development of your child towards normal, healthy growth. After your baby is born, you will be rewarded 100 times over.

Some time ago physicians thought that inside the womb the unborn child was well protected against toxins. Now we know that this was only wishful thinking and that many toxins can pass through the placenta into the unborn child. Maybe, originally, the placenta really was a dependable barrier against toxins, but since our environment has been drastically altered, that is not the case any more. New and formerly unknown so-called 'food' has taken the place of 'no-nonsense', plain, nutritious meals and our living habits have taken a turn for the worse. Since the chemical deluge began several built-in defence mechanisms of our body have been damaged and do not function properly any longer. Even in the earliest weeks of pregnancy the poisons from tobacco, drugs and food additives can pass through the barrier of the placenta and endanger the unborn child. Alcohol and the nicotine in cigarettes may distort the developing nerve cells of the baby. As well as alcohol and nicotine, coffee, black tea, sugary drinks, sweets, unhealthy snacks and junk food can harm the embryo and might influence not only its physical, but also its mental development. The state of health of the mother during this time is vitally important for the child. Whatever happens, good or bad, during the period of pregnancy has an effect upon a child that will last for the rest of its life. If the expectant mother pollutes her internal biochemistry with drugs, alcohol, nicotine or even caffeine, she is poisoning the environment of her child. The child is exposed to these toxins for nine months.

We know, for example, that babies born to women who smoke during pregnancy usually have a lower intelligence quotient than many other babies. Amalgam (mercury, alloyed with several other metals) from dental fillings or from mercury-contaminated fish is a nerve poison that can cause a miscarriage or foetal deformities. Lead and hundreds of other substances from the exhaust fumes of cars or factories can harm the foetus and affect its nervous and immune system. Wherever possible the use of tranquillisers, diuretic or stimulant drugs and amphetamine-containing appetite suppressants should be avoided during pregnancy. Mental deficiencies, hyperactivity, infantile autism, learning disabilities and other behaviour disorders seem to be closely related to bad eating habits and the use of certain drugs by the future mother, including some medication for the relief of nausea and vomiting, or sedatives. If you really think you need medication, do not buy it over the counter. Instead, talk it over with an understanding and open-minded physician. Almost all prescription and over-the-counter drugs that suppress symptoms are dangerous for future mothers and their babies. It is very important to choose the right kind of physician and you should not just go to anyone, even if he or she is a well-known and important professor. Sometimes such a title does not mean much; it only shows that the doctor studied longer, and has perhaps written some interesting papers and books. However, this does not prove that such doctors know more than a regular physician, and often they have less practical experience. The old and beloved family doctor often knew the entire family and all their problems and really could help when needed. Sadly, this kind of doctor is almost extinct now.

Medical doctors should give a good example by looking healthy themselves; they should not be too fat, smoke or drink much alcohol, and above all they should not prescribe strong drugs, except in an emergency. They should take enough time with their patients and give sound advice, which is far more important than just writing a prescription.

Prospective mothers should now be able to prevent some of the health problems that might threaten their unborn children because most of the facts about such dangers are known. However, the health education of the general public is far behind the times and there are still many things we cannot foresee or prevent. Knowledge about all the possible dangers is extremely important, so I will bring you up to date as much as possible with the facts. Day by day the technical and chemical pollution of our planet is increasing and there are many dangers we are hardly aware of. When you are expecting a baby it is high time for you to realise what is going on, so that you can steer clear of threats to your child's health.

When a woman is expecting a child enormous changes take place in her body. Her metabolism, hormones and immune system have to adapt in order to make it possible for the new life in her to grow and develop. In our Western countries many women suffer from morning sickness in the first three months of pregnancy. This is because of a lack of adaptation to metabolic changes in the body. Why does this happen mainly in industrial countries? It is because we eat the wrong kind of food. Because of this our blood sugar is often too low, there is a lack of hydrochloric acid and probably also a lack of B vitamins. Most things we eat induce an acid reaction and because our organism wants to get rid of this surplus of acidity, we have the urge to vomit. Millions of women have low blood sugar and are nervous, depressed, irritable, overtired and suffer from nausea and vomiting. Animals, and people still living in a natural habitat and leading a healthy life, do not have such problems.

Thousands of years ago, famous physicians were of the opinion that most diseases start in our intestines. Now many people have realised that the old doctors were right. When expecting a baby, our nutrition must be more than merely adequate; it must be the best that circumstances allow. Bad eating habits of the mother are amongst the most important causal factors of uncountable diseases and behaviour problems of future children. Every cell in our body needs the right nutrients in order to function in an optimal way and our brain needs about one-third of our daily nutrient intake. When some important nutrients are missing, many cells weaken or even die.

The mother's habits during the nine-month period of pregnancy have a lasting effect upon the child. Sometimes, because of ignorance or lack of intelligence, a future mother may endanger the health of her child without realising it. Junk food is lacking in vitamins and other nutrients that children need in order to develop a healthy body and mind. The eating habits of some young women can be so bad that their babies are barely kept alive. Wrong eating and living habits while conceiving and bearing a child can all too often mean the destruction of happiness for everyone concerned. It is a great joy and much less work to care for a healthy baby. The best guarantee of having a healthy baby is to be healthy yourself.

Women who do not understand these things often deliver children that are unable to cope with life. The punishment for such neglect is severe, because it is very difficult to care for an ailing child. A lack of proper nutrients, in adequate amounts, can produce deficiencies with catastrophic consequences in a child.

Not until the past decade of research was it learned that during the prenatal period human beings are more susceptible to the environment than they will ever be again in their lives. Dr Alfred Tomatis, a specialist in ear, nose and throat diseases and professor in audio-psycho-phonology in Paris, is known as the pioneer of music and sound therapy, as well as of prenatal psychology. His best-known book, *La Nuit Uterine* (*Night in the Uterus*), is beautifully written and very interesting. Professor Tomatis describes how more and more scientists have come to the conclusion that in the first nine months of our life the foundations of our personality, for example our ability to think, feel and express ourselves, and our self-confidence, are being moulded.

He explains that the ear of the embryo develops much faster than the other organs. (The word 'embryo' is used during the first nine weeks; thereafter the human embryo is called a 'foetus'.) The development of the human ear starts very early, more or less after 22 days of pregnancy and after about four months the foetus can hear the voices of its parents and can differentiate between high and low, harmonious and discordant sounds. Sound waves are energy waves and Dr Tomatis explains in his book that these energy waves resound in the brain and their radiation influences the rest of the organism of the foetus. They are a basic necessity for the further development of the foetus.

In Austria there was a wonderful lady doctor working in one of the big hospitals in Vienna. This doctor was extremely successful in keeping babies alive that were born very prematurely. She let the mother keep her baby with her after birth and used music therapy. Guess what? She was not permitted to work in the hospital any longer, because such treatment was not 'officially recognised'.

Noise pollution is a very serious problem in foetal development and researchers now know that too much noise brings chaos into all our lives. The radio might be blaring, the television on, the phone ringing and the children yelling at the top of their voices. This cacophony of noise, which is a real strain even for our ears and the ears of teenagers used to loud music, must be a terrible stress on the very sensitive, tiny ears of a foetus. Harmonious, nice music on the other hand stimulates positive development in the foetus; harsh and unharmonious sounds are dangerous and could possibly impair normal physical and mental growth. One of the worst things a pregnant woman could do is go to a festival of rock music, as her unborn baby would be forced to listen for several hours to hard, unharmonious sounds. By doing so she would risk damaging her future child for life.

Later in pregnancy other senses start developing. Formerly it was thought that eating habits were formed in the first years of life, but recently there has been much research that seems to confirm that the development of certain likes and dislikes of foods are already being determined during foetal development. Children may develop likes or dislikes their mother had during pregnancy. This is another reason why pregnant women should have healthy eating habits.

❧ Chapter 4 ❧

BREAST-FEEDING YOUR BABY

After your baby is born and the doctor has assured you that everything went well, and that your baby is fine, it will be your greatest wish that your baby will always be healthy and happy. Health has nothing to do with luck, but it has much to do with healthy parents and a good measure of intelligence, knowledge, willpower and faith in your personal judgement.

When expecting your baby, you will have had plenty of time to read and learn all about pregnancy and how to take care of your baby. The most important thing is to decide how to feed it; your choice will influence the health of your child for the rest of its life.

Nowadays the number of paediatricians that recommend breast-feeding is growing. It is really a shame that for many years about 75 per cent of all newborn babies did not receive their mother's milk. However, thank God, now there are again more mothers insisting on breast-feeding.

At university, medical students are taught hardly anything about nutrition and only a few physicians realise that the right nutrition is one of the most important things in life, especially in the life of newborn babies. Many doctors are men, who have perhaps had the chance to bottle-feed a baby once in a while at the most. About breast-feeding they know very little as, of course, they have no personal experience in doing this.

Breast-feeding your baby is the natural thing to do and it is the best health insurance you can give your child. However, bottle-feeding gives you more freedom, as other people can also bottle-feed your baby. But whatever the doctor tells you, industrially prepared baby food is always a risk and both the baby and the mother need the personal contact that comes with breast-feeding.

Infant formulas made with a base of cow's milk contain almost three times as much protein as human milk. This puts a great strain on a baby's kidneys. In all respects cow's milk is completely different milk from human milk and is difficult to digest – not for a calf, but for a human baby.

Babies fed with cow's milk weigh more than babies who are breast-fed; we say that they have 'baby fat'. This is not a sign of health, but that the small kidneys of your baby retain too much fluid and their tissues have become waterlogged. This is a defensive measure the body takes in order to prevent kidney damage.

If you took care of your health during pregnancy and did nothing stupid like taking amphetamines, tranquillisers or diuretic drugs, there is a good chance that your children will be healthy – you have given them the right foundations. The second step is to give them the building materials needed for the healthy development of their bodies and minds.

In almost all families there are traces of inheritable diseases, but unless these are very serious, there is no need to worry. If your baby gets the right nutrition and care, in most cases the genes of such diseases will stay dormant and have no opportunity to develop and break out. However, if the defence mechanisms of your baby are damaged through bad nutrition and other negative factors, inherited diseases might develop.

As a consequence of the general pollution of our environment and of our daily food, every year there are more children suffering not only from physical but also from mental diseases. Never before have there been so many children suffering from symptoms such as restlessness, aggressive behaviour, apathy, depression, anti-social behaviour, attention deficit disorders, allergies, minimal brain dysfunction, hyperactivity, autism and others. Some of these problems might even start during pregnancy, or right after. This is very worrying, but if you have a bad conscience because you neglected your health during pregnancy and feel terribly sorry about it, you might still be able to remedy any damage to your children by giving them all they need for good health from now on – do not despair.

However, it is important to realise what might happen if a very sensitive little baby gets exposed to indigestible or toxic food, or to any other type of neglect.

As soon as babies have one or two teeth they can have something more solid than milk. In the chemist's or even the health-food shop you will find very attractive and appetising-looking little jars of baby food. However, little babies need natural food and not food from jars, as you never know what these may contain. Although such products from the health-food shop usually do not contain any chemical preservatives, they must be able to be stored for a long time and so they will have been treated by heat or other means. One of the biggest producers of baby food (Gerber Baby Foods) claimed that all their baby food was natural. However, in 1997 there was a lawsuit against the firm, because it could be proved that several of its products contained preservatives. Therefore, my advice is not to buy any manufactured baby food, even if it claims to be 'natural'; take the trouble to make the food for your baby at home. Buying baby food in jars is good for the producer, but not for the baby. Babies and toddlers need fresh food, prepared preferably right before they eat it. Please, never reheat any baby food, as this is not advisable for your baby's health.

Both parents have to realise that having a child is an enormous responsibility, but young people are often too frightened, too unsure of themselves and too weak-willed to do the right thing. In order to be able to take care of a child you need to be grown-up yourself, and you should have the strength of character and necessary patience to do what is best for the child and give proper guidance.

The following story will demonstrate the kind of problems many young parents can encounter. Peggy had been married for five years and when she discovered she was pregnant, she and her husband were delighted. They were not very young any more and had almost given up hope of ever having a child. Besides some minor complications during the birth of little Sandra, mother and child were doing fine. The only problem was that Peggy could not feed her baby. After the birth she was very nervous, as she had almost no milk. Nobody had told her that this was normal, as the breast often only gives milk after several days. Peggy did not know this and soon decided to give up on breast-feeding. This was a pity, but fortunately the baby took to the bottle without any problems and seemed to be happy and healthy.

However, after a few months Peggy noticed that from time to time Sandra would perspire profusely, even when the room was rather cool. She also often cried for a long time and nothing her parents did helped; she was inconsolable. Sometimes her little tummy felt blown up and seemed to be full of gas. The family physician changed the bottle formula several times and, at last, found a formula that seemed to be better. Then the crying spells would start anew and often end in temper tantrums. After such a tantrum little Sandra would be completely washed out and dead tired. Sometimes she was very affectionate and clingy, and at other times she turned her head when her parents wanted to pet or kiss her.

By the time the baby was one year old, she only had her baby formula once or twice a day and she loved to eat the different baby foods that her mother bought in the chemist's. However, Sandra's tantrums had not stopped and she became even more restless. She could not keep still for one moment and was in constant motion. Whenever her mother tried to calm her down she started yelling at the top of her voice. Often she tried to destroy her toys or her dolls. The situation became quite chaotic; both parents had come to their wits' end and went to see a child psychiatrist. This doctor suggested giving Sandra a light tranquilliser and it did indeed help, but whenever they stopped giving her the drugs the symptoms came right back and were even worse.

Peggy and her husband had heard about the clinic of Dr Pfeiffer near New York. The physicians there specialised in helping parents and their children in unorthodox ways, with a high degree of success. Peggy and her husband took their little daughter to this clinic, where the doctors gave her a very thorough check-up. These physicians found that the child was allergic to cows' milk, as well as to wheat, and lacked certain vitamins. They recommended that little Sandra should eat no more industrially prepared food and prescribed a diet with lots of fresh vegetables, as well as high quantities of vitamin B3 and other vitamins. Sandra's mother followed this to the letter and by the time she was three years old, the child had changed into a lovely and very healthy little girl.

Although there are still many women who do not want to take the time or trouble to feed their babies in the natural way, fortunately breast-feeding is once again gaining popularity in industrial countries. There are some excellent organisations helping women with problems in this respect, such as 'La Lêche League', an international organisation that was founded in Canada. This organisation is very successful and is based on the belief that mothers should help each other.

The ideal nutrition for a newborn baby is its mother's milk. Breast milk contains all the nutrients needed for the healthy development of the body as well as the brain of a baby, and its natural antibodies strengthen and activate the baby's immune system. As long as a mother breast-feeds her baby there is little danger of the child getting infections or a disease. When expecting a baby every future mother should learn some important things about breast-feeding. Because of a lack of knowledge, the new mother might be so nervous that feeding her baby becomes a problem and the milk flow never really gets going or even stops altogether. Knowledge about all the facts concerning breast-feeding is the best defence a mother has against physicians who are in a hurry, or well-meaning nurses who may have never had a baby themselves and recommend giving a bottle. A patient and loving mother should always enjoy her baby, and should not be distracted by needless anxiety or the interference of others.

The colostrum (fore-milk) is the first concentrated milk from the human breast. It contains all the special nutrients a newborn baby needs and during the first days, the baby needs only a few drops of it once in a while. Babies still have plenty of reserve supplies of nutrients from their nine-month stay in the womb, and it does not matter at all if this is the only food they take for the first couple of days. Do not worry if even after two or three days your breast hardly gives any milk. Your baby is not yet really hungry, and does not suck hard enough to stimulate the milk flow. Patience and love are the most important factors for a new mother and her baby. Just put your baby to the breast for a little while until it gets tired and when it wakes up, try again on the other breast and so on, until it starts sucking properly. Once babies really start to suck, they will suck harder each time and the harder they suck, the more milk will flow. That is the way of nature, and you and your baby are an integral part of it. By instinct you will know what is best for both of you.

Babies live in your body for a whole nine months, so they have heard your voice and trust you. Babies must be kept close to their mothers as much as possible; they will suck, but in their own time, when they are ready for it and not before. Do not let anybody force you or your baby. There is no better place for newborn babies than on the tummy of their mother, or right next to her.

However, while mothers are still in hospital some nurses may try to give their babies a bottle without their knowledge, and may even use a little sugar or honey to make it more attractive. Such a nurse probably means well, but nurses can spoil babies that way; they will not want to suck at the breast any more, as it is much harder work. If this happens, however, do not worry. The problem can usually be solved as soon as you are back home. Put the bottle away in a dark corner, and put your baby on your tummy. Take the time to get it used to your breast. Never force your baby and allow it to sleep if it wants to. As I have said, it may take a couple of days before the child really starts sucking, but babies always get more food than you think, and they really need very little. Babies are like little animals: their will to survive is extremely strong and going hungry for a few days will not hurt them at all. Of course, they might lose a little weight, but within a few days or a week they will suck harder than ever and make up for it. If you understand this and support your baby, everything will be fine and you will feel a deep happiness spreading through you. All the trouble and time you have been spending with your baby will have been worthwhile.

Breast-feeding is a great joy and gives both mother and child a wonderful feeling of contentment. Once you start breast-feeding, you will develop a great relationship that in later years will help you to understand your child. At every stage, the quality and composition of the milk the baby receives changes automatically; its composition adapts to the ever-changing needs of the child.

As long as you are breast-feeding your baby it is very important to refrain from drinking coffee, black tea, alcohol, soft drinks or anything else that could hurt the child. Always remember that whatever you eat or drink goes into your milk and can affect your infant. What does not hurt you may hurt babies, as they are far more sensitive then you are. If you eat or drink something that does not agree with your baby you will soon know it, for it will show signs of not feeling well: a rash, vomiting too often (a little bit is quite normal), constipation or a change in bowel movements.

In order to find out what has caused the problem, you will have to be a good detective. Usually, breast-fed babies give little trouble and much happiness. This happy state often changes as soon as they are given the bottle. Bottle-feeding is not nearly as personal as breast-feeding. Now is the time when problems may start. Quiet and friendly babies, who used to fall asleep when their tummies were full, may now suffer from gases or aches and sometimes cry for a long time. They may get a nappy rash and not sleep so well any more. Doctors usually say that the formula such babies are being given does not agree with them, and prescribe another. Some paediatricians are in the habit of changing these formulas regularly, but often they never seem to find the right one. To be honest, it stands to reason that babies do not thrive on any of these formulas; they are human beings and not calves.

Every kind of animal milk has been designed for its own kind: little lambs drink sheep's milk, foals drink horses' milk and piglets drink pigs' milk. In the milk of its mother every animal finds the nutrients that are exactly adapted to its special needs, and in every kind of milk the nutrients are completely different. Cows' milk is deficient in iron. It contains almost three times as much protein as human milk and it is a different kind of protein. Although cows' milk contains much calcium, magnesium and other goodies, the calcium and other nutrients are in quality and quantity different from the same nutrients in human milk. They are meant for baby cows and their special requirements. No wonder that many babies, children and adults never get used to drinking cows' milk.

Some people, even physicians, advise pregnant or nursing women to drink milk and eat plenty of milk products while expecting and feeding a baby. According to these people, a cow should also drink plenty of milk in order to be able to produce milk. If you look at the big, strong bones of a cow, you may wonder where she gets her calcium from. A cow gets her calcium in wintertime from hay and in summer, when she gives her best milk, from green grass, plants and fresh herbs. Likewise, the best sources of calcium for human beings do not come from milk or milk products, but from vegetables, fruits, roots, nuts and dried fruit.

Perhaps your baby will get used to drinking cows' milk – some babies do, and look very healthy as they have more so-called 'baby-fat' than breast-fed babies.

However, 'fat' does not mean 'healthy'. Bottle-feeding with infant formulas often predisposes babies to lifelong obesity. Lean, breast-fed infants usually have more resistance to disease, and their brain develops faster than the brain of bottle-fed babies. Sometimes it is really not possible for mothers to feed their babies themselves, but if cows' milk does not agree with your baby you should never insist that it drinks it; it might really do some harm.

Soya milk was the big fashion some years ago. For several reasons, however, except once in a while, soya milk is also not the ideal food for your baby. There are many other kinds of milk that contain calcium and other important nutrients. You can buy these in a health-food shop, or preferably prepare them at home. Using nuts, almonds, sunflower and other seeds, or even wholemeal cereals or rice, you can make wonderful baby milk. Fill the glass of a mixer with natural mineral water (unfizzy, of course!) halfway up and add a handful of one of these foods. Mix this for a few minutes and then strain through a fine sieve. You will have to experiment with these vegetable milk drinks. Please remember never to add sugar or even honey to them. Sugar is one of the most health-damaging products there is and as babies do not yet have a sweet tooth like grown-ups, you should not get them used to the taste. You can save yourself and your child a lot of problems in this way.

The later they discover sugar, the longer children will stay in good health.

Whenever you give your baby a new type of vegetable milk, start with a spoonful at a time and if there is no adverse reaction, increase the quantity gradually. It is important that you change the diet of your baby once in a while so that he receives all the different vitamins and minerals he needs.

After some months, besides breast milk and vegetable milk, young children can gradually start eating grated fruit, like apples, mashed boiled carrots or potatoes, and other soft fruit and vegetables. As soon as the first teeth appear, milk slowly stops being a natural food for babies. The composition of the digestive juices change, and babies become little toddlers and need different foods. Slowly you should wean them from the breast; this will be no problem, as at that stage milk does not appeal as much as before.

This is not a book about baby food. You will find quite a few good cookbooks for baby food in the shops. In this chapter I only wanted to emphasise the importance of giving your child good, healthy food; it is one of the best means of preventing diseases of the body and the mind, and prevent the heartbreaking experience of having a mentally or emotionally disturbed child.

✌ Chapter 5 ✌

BREAST-FEEDING AND WET-NURSES

For thousands of years breast-feeding a baby was the only option. If the mother died or was unable to breast-feed, the baby would not survive unless another woman could be found who would do so. Later on, in Egypt, in the Roman Empire and in Greece, royalty, nobility and important merchants used wet-nurses for the convenience of their ladies, who had many social commitments. (Read the beautiful story of Halimah later in this chapter.)

Maybe you recall the story of the twins, Romulus and Remus, who were the mythical founders of Rome. They were placed in a basket at birth and set afloat on the Tiber. The basket came aground under a fig tree where they were suckled by a she-wolf. Of course, in real life people also tried to use substitutes for human milk. Wolves' milk was not available, so they used cows' or goats' milk, which was drunk from sucking horns and other receptacles. However, most babies who drank animal milk did not seem to thrive and often became ill or even died.

In the Middle Ages wet-nurses were 'in' and many more people made use of their services. Then, between 1600 and 1900 there was a protest movement from 'modern' mothers who preferred to nurse their own babies again. Around that time so-called 'dry-nursing' also became fashionable, because it was much cheaper than employing a wet-nurse. Dry-nursing meant making a kind of porridge from flour, cereals and water. However, babies often became constipated with this kind of food or had belly-aches.

Although in the twentieth century most woman in rural areas

were still breast-feeding their offspring, in the cities more and more women were buying the new breast-milk substitutes that appeared in growing quantities on the market.

However, in the beginning especially the quality of these products left much to be desired and many babies became ill – mortality was high. Baby food soon became big business and without it many more children would probably have died. However, these substitutes, based on cows' milk, can never be compared to the real thing. These companies are trying all the time to improve their formulas so that they resemble human milk as much as possible, and are always inventing new ways to manipulate their product.

The milk of a cow is originally a 'living food' that contains many valuable nutrients for calves. In a factory this milk has to be subjected to very high temperatures, whereby most proteins and nutrients are destroyed. When the temperature of our own body is over 43 degrees the same thing happens to us; in that case proteins coagulate and our body cells die. Babies can only be really healthy when they receive 'living food' from their own mothers. After heating, baby milk undergoes many changes. With each manipulation more of the valuable nutrients of the original living product are lost. A baby formula is a dead product. If they are fed it, babies will grow and be kept alive, but that is about all. Babies brought up with the bottle will never be as healthy as breast-fed babies and will never have the same kind of self-defence mechanisms, which in our time are so badly needed. More babies all the time are unable to digest cows' milk or are allergic to it. Infant formulas have been produced in such a way that they smell and taste good to a baby and its parents, but in no way can these ever be compared to human milk.

HALIMAH: THE WET-NURSE Adapted from *Mahjubah Magazine,* February, 1987

In the history of Islam, many women have made themselves known due to their courage, valour and inspiring faith. Some of them have earned renown because of their brave deeds and exemplary Islamic behaviour. However, some have had honour bestowed upon them solely through the grace of Almighty Allah, who saw fit to single them out with a divine reward.

One such personality was Halimah, a great lady from the respectable Arab tribe of Bani Sa'di. Halimah was divinely chosen from among many pure and honourable women to be the wet-nurse of the Seal of the Prophets, Muhammad. The noble mother of Muhammad died shortly after the birth of the Prophet, which left him a young infant, without the benefits of being suckled and nursed by a mother. Muhammad's father at that time was on a journey and so he was left in the custody of his grandfather, Abdul Mutaleb. His grandfather was searching Mecca to find a mother to nurse the young hungry infant.

Divine destiny intervened at that time: Halimah and a group of other women were travelling to Mecca. A very severe famine and drought in the region of the Bani Sa'di had forced the women, all mothers with nursing infants, to travel to Mecca seeking jobs as wet-nurses. Halimah herself related the amazing story of how she came to be chosen as the wet-nurse to feed the infant who was to become the most noble Messenger of Allah, Seal of the Prophets.

> We were travelling towards Mecca on donkeys and camels, hoping to find jobs nursing suckling infants. The drought and famine had left us all hungry and poverty stricken. Our farms had become barren and our animals sick and worthless.
>
> I was riding on a very slow, tired donkey, cradling an infant of my own who had to go to sleep hungry at nights since my milk was not enough to satisfy him. I hoped that maybe if I found a job as a wet-nurse our poverty may be slightly alleviated.
>
> When we arrived in Mecca, Abdul Mutaleb had asked the women to take Muhammad but no one accepted because since he was an orphan they thought they wouldn't be paid well enough. However his grandfather didn't give up and continued to ask other women if they would accept the infant Muhammad. I decided to offer my help to Abdul Mutaleb and I told him I was able to accept his infant. He asked me who I was and I told him, 'I am Halimah from the tribe of Bani Sa'di.' He smiled and said, 'You are from a tribe

which is renowned for being fortunate (*saadar*) and your name is Halimah, which means patient. These qualities are rewarded in this world and the next.'

He agreed to give me Muhammad and took me to the home of Aminah the mother of Muhammad. As soon as I laid eyes on the baby I fell in love with his beautiful, yet strangely noble face. I took hold of him and cradled him in my arms. Without any encouragement he immediately took to my breast and began feeding. However, no matter what I did he wouldn't take milk from my right breast. He always only fed from the left one and in this way I was able to feed my own infant from my right breast.

I took Muhammad back with me to my own home, and amazingly my breasts became so full of milk that I was able to feed both my own child and Muhammad. I felt a strange sense of elation while nursing Muhammad. Despite being weak and undernourished, with hardly enough milk to fill one small child, I was suddenly producing enough milk to satiate two hungry infants. But the divine benefits bestowed on us didn't stop there.

From the moment we brought the child Muhammad into our home we were bestowed with successive fortune. Our sheep and camels became fat and healthy, our farm flourished. We were miraculously spared any disease that befell the animals of our neighbours. Nursing and caring for Muhammad was so pleasurable that I soon regarded him with just as much love and affection as my own children.

When Muhammad reached five years of age, he asked me one morning where his brothers went every day. I told him that they took the sheep to graze in the nearby hills. Muhammad insisted that he accompany his brothers that morning, so I allowed him to go. After a while one of my sons returned saying, 'They have taken Muhammad.' Quickly I went to the hills and there I found Muhammad alone, but it seemed that a dazzling light engulfed him. I embraced him and asked what had happened. He calmly answered 'Mother Halimah, don't worry, God is with me.'

Halimah experienced so many other strange and divine incidents during Muhammad's childhood that she was left in no doubt about the uniqueness of the orphan divine fate had led her to choose to bring up. She herself was of course of a special purity, so that Almighty Allah selected her to nurse his Seal of the Prophets. Her efforts and troubles in lovingly bringing up Muhammad would no doubt be rewarded in the next world.

HOW TO FEED YOUR BABY OR TODDLER

Under exactly the same circumstances, the behaviour of babies can be totally different. Even a small baby already has its personality and this shows early in life. After only a few months a mother knows right away when there is a change in the behaviour of her baby, and she will try to find out what the cause could be. For babies who are bottle-fed especially, this might be a blown-up tummy, a nappy rash, sneezing spells, vomiting or dozens of other things. However, so long as the vomiting is not too severe and the baby eats and sleeps well, some vomiting is completely normal. Some babies suck too hard and bottle-fed babies often tend to drink more than they really need. Sometimes there is not enough room in their tummy and they react by throwing up the surplus milk. Babies can be just as greedy as grown-up people.

However, if your baby cries or even screams for a long time (especially after meals), sleeps badly during the night, has constipation or loses too much weight, there really might be something wrong with its food. In that case you should consult a good paediatrician who knows about homoeopathy and natural treatments, and above all about the right kind of food for babies. It still amazes me that there are so few paediatricians and other doctors who really know about food, but at university, even for future paediatricians, nutrition is, and for a long time has been, a subject of minor importance.

Even at a very tender age, the wrong kind of nutrition can be the direct or indirect cause of all kinds of diseases, now and in later life, and every mother should learn about what is healthy for her baby or toddler. Do not buy industrial baby food in nice little containers or jars, prepared in factories. Buying such food might save you some work in the kitchen now, but later when your baby falls ill, you will have ten times more work. It is so easy to prepare vegetable milk (see page 36) or prepare a fresh vegetable mash at home.

Even when babies are still small, you should look out for any food allergies or incompatibilities. Never force babies or toddlers to eat. Their instinctive reactions are still very good and they usually know when their tummies are full or when something does not agree with them. At an early age some babies or small children may already be allergic to certain foods (such as tomatoes, potatoes, wheat and others). If children refuse to eat something, just take their bottles or plates away and prepare something different next time. Do not give them anything to eat for some hours. Refusing to eat may just be a way to attract your attention, and you will soon find out if it is. Little children can be devils sometimes, although they may look like angels.

Small pieces of fruit or grated vegetables can be a nice meal for a toddler; they really need very little food when they are tiny. The size of their stomach is about the size of their closed fist and if you look at how small the fist is, you will realise that your child probably does not need all the food you serve him. If children like eating and are given too much food at every meal, their stomachs will stretch out and become too big. Their tummies are like something made from elastic. If an elastic band is over-stretched a few times, it goes back into shape, but if this happens constantly the elastic becomes weak and loses its characteristics. When this happens to the tummy of a child it is not good at all. Such a big tummy needs to be filled all the time and the child gets used to eating too much. Loving mothers giving their children too much to eat often causes them to be fat and unhealthy. Such children will not be happy. There is a Japanese proverb that says: 'If you love your child, beat him; if you hate your child, give him much to eat.' Although I am definitely against beating a child, I agree completely with the second part of this proverb. Children should enjoy eating, but too much food can do a lot of harm.

Find out what your children like – healthy food that agrees with them. Never let them get used to having soft drinks, sweets, chips or other salty stuff. Such 'non-food' gives them an enormous amount of calories and takes away their appetites completely. Too much salt will ruin their kidneys. If a child gets used to these things, it will soon become very sick. Thanks to soft drinks and junk food, there are thousands of children who are listless, pale, hyperactive or very nervous and suffer from chronic colds, earaches and many other trivial, or even serious diseases.

&❧ Chapter 7 ❧&

AGGRESSIVE TODDLERS

It happens more and more often that kindergartens refuse to take small children who bite, slap and fight with other children. Some babies may even show signs of aggressiveness, biting their mothers' breasts. As soon as they are a bit older they will also bite their brothers and sisters whenever they have the opportunity. In kindergarten they are feared, not only because of their aggressiveness, but also because they love to destroy things and nothing is safe when they are around.

When talking with the parents of such children, they often tell me that their children were darling babies who gave no trouble at all. Then out of the blue everything changed. Their sweet baby started to cry for hours on end and became a little devil. In medical practices we often hear the same stories.

These children can seem to change their entire personalities within a few weeks and at the same time start suffering from all kinds of health problems, like nappy rashes, scaly skin, runny noses, allergies, sleeplessness and so on. Sometimes parents worry too much. There is usually nothing serious the matter, and their children recover quickly. It is quite natural for small children to be wild, exited, nervous and aggressive once in a while and they may become almost unmanageable for days or weeks. Even for us grown-ups it is not always easy to cope with life; just imagine what children have to get used to when growing up. Their small worlds suddenly become bigger and they have to tackle new and often frightening problems. Fortunately some children remain well balanced, trusting and calm. But many do not adapt so easily. They become nervous and easily frightened, and those are the children who often become aggressive. However, when children hardly react at all and seem to withdraw into themselves it is not a good sign at all. Such children need much love and understanding. This kind of behaviour can be temporary, and may be due to something that has made them terribly unhappy. In that case you will have to find out what is the matter and then reassure and help them in a loving way until they find their inner peace again.

Do not worry too much – your child is probably perfectly normal. But when children sleep only for a few hours each night instead of the eight, ten or more hours they need, often yell or scream for a long time, destroy their own toys and those of other children, or bite, scratch and slap anybody who dares to cross their path, there is definitely something wrong.

A happy family life is not possible when a child has terrible tantrums, never sits still for one moment and behaves like a mad little dog. Then there is no peace in the house.

Here is a story one of my patients told me.

PAT'S STORY

What a great feeling it was after nine months of pregnancy to hold such a beautiful tiny baby in my arms. I felt so happy I cried for joy. For the first couple of months everything was fine. The baby had a good appetite and after filling his belly at my breast, he fell asleep almost immediately. He slept for many hours, so that my husband and I most of the time also had a good night's sleep.

My baby was so easy to handle, and my husband and I did not really believe it, when other parents told us about all the problems they had with their offspring. We enjoyed being parents; life was good and our baby hardly gave us any trouble.

After five months of breast-feeding, I started giving my baby a bottle once a day. The formula was based on cows' milk and my doctor recommended a special brand. Tasting cows' milk for the first time, my son made a face, but he got used to it pretty soon. Sometimes he cried after finishing his bottle and I had the feeling he was still hungry.

When his first teeth came through I had not yet stopped breast-feeding him altogether. One day when he started to cry and I put him to my breast I got quite a shock, because he suddenly bit me. It hurt a lot and now it was my turn to cry. After that time he bit me more often. At that time he did not sleep longer than two or three hours in a row. He was extremely restless and often cried for a long time. After weeks of this my husband and I became very tired and sometimes we fought, which had never happened before.

I stopped breast-feeding my son altogether and as well as his bottle gave him baby food from jars. He was not a sweet baby any more at all. He bit my hand or my arm whenever he had a chance. Happiness went out of the window and as he kept attacking me I even became a little afraid of my own child. I wondered why, and imagined that maybe I had done something wrong and my baby did not love me any more. My husband said it came from his family; his brother had also been very aggressive as a child and we all knew that later on this brother had to be put in an asylum. It was a family secret and they were all ashamed that this had happened in their family.

I insisted that my baby was not insane, and I really believed it was my own fault; maybe I had not shown him enough love. We went with our child to many doctors, who did their best, but in the end they gave up and sent us to a children's psychiatrist. In the course of a year this doctor prescribed different tranquillisers, but these only made things worse. My son seemed to sleep all the time now: sometimes he woke up all of a sudden and for short periods he became more aggressive than ever before.

Then we started reading about hyperactivity, autism, depression, schizophrenia and other mental problems and diseases. We heard about wonderful physicians like Dr Ben

Feingold, Dr Pfeiffer, Dr Richard Mackarnes and others. Although these doctors used unorthodox ways of treatment, they were very successful in treating mentally ill and/or disturbed patients, so we realised that there was still hope for our baby. We gave it a try and with their help our child became again the sweet and healthy child he originally was.

Apart from the influence a happy or an unhappy home life has on a child and aside from how much or how little love and understanding a child receives, the environment of almost all children born in our time has changed so much that it is no wonder many children have physical or mental problems.

People who haven't any children themselves have not the faintest idea about all the things that may happen at home or at school nowadays. There are parents and teachers who are absolutely desperate, and newspapers and magazines from France to China have published several very alarming articles about the inefficiency and impotency of our educational systems. Often children have seized control. Teachers and parents are just the onlookers, and seem to be helpless. Only a few people seem to understand what really is happening.

ஒ Chapter 8 ஒ

CHILDREN WITH LEARNING DISABILITIES

In the last two or three decades the increase in the number of children with learning difficulties has been considerable. A growing percentage of non-retarded, often very intelligent, children in the United States and Europe suffer from dyslexia or dysgraphia. Dyslexia means that a child has trouble understanding written words, sentences or paragraphs. Dysgraphia means that it is hard for a child to form letters or write within a defined space. Although there are other learning problems, these two are the most common.

In the UK there are about one million children with learning problems; in the United States probably five or six times as many. Often learning disabilities (LD) are associated with Attention Deficit/Hyperactive Disorder (AD/HD) or other behavioural problems. In school, many of these kids try to divert attention from their handicap by erratic and bad behaviour. Small boys may jump up and down pulling faces, and girls may start crying or even screaming. When they get older, their frustrations are expressed in different ways that may be even worse.

Most of these children are very unhappy and miserable, because they do not understand why learning is so difficult for them, while for other children it seems to be easy. Other children might tease them or hold them up to ridicule. Children can be very cruel and consequently the problems intensify.

They may be accused of laziness or attention-seeking, or their parents may be blamed for their behaviour. But most parents feel helpless and sometimes desperate; educating their children seems to be an impossible task. They do not understand their children and they cannot reach them. Such children can disrupt relationships and destroy family life. The divorce rate of their parents is high, and this is disastrous for the children's future.

Some physicians believe that the cause is a malfunctioning of one area of the brain. This might be induced by physical damage to the brain, but such damage can seldom be proved, except when there has been asphyxia (lack of oxygen) during birth. Furthermore, most AD/HD children and children with learning problems have a high intelligence quotient and in my opinion this erases brain damage as a possible cause.

When a child has difficulty in learning or writing, the first thing that needs to be done is a test for possible visual or hearing problems. Sometimes children do not even know what the teacher is talking about because their hearing is far below average, or they cannot see what is written on the blackboard because of bad eyesight. Each of these children should have an eye examination performed by a specialist in vision development. Such a physician investigates the function of the eyes as well as their structure. The hearing of these children should also be thoroughly checked, and sometimes it is wonderful to observe how much these children improve on all levels as soon as their vision or hearing is dealt with. Often children's personalities seem to change from one day to another when their feelings of inferiority disappear and their self-esteem goes up. Although hyperactive children may always be somewhat restless and impulsive, there is no more need for them to disrupt the order of an entire classroom because they feel so terribly unsure of themselves.

Unfortunately it is not always that easy. Children suffering from AD/HD and learning deficiencies often suffer from recurring infections, like ear infections (*otitis media*) or rhinitis. Most of the time these infections are treated symptomatically with antibiotics and therefore never have a chance to really heal up. The toxins of these masked and hidden chronic infections enter the general bloodstream day by day and add to the general toxicity of an already diseased organism. Because of an allergic disposition and as a consequence of the regular influx of toxins, many children suffer from asthma, eczema, digestive disturbances, gas, diarrhoea or constipation. This merry-go-round never ends until the patient is treated by a physician who understands the natural connections of everything that happens in the human body. There are few physicians or laymen who understand that improper food-body-brain interactions, sustained by habitual food choices, produce the patterns of dysfunction commonly observed.

Many children are fussy eaters and the first foods refused are vegetables, often in favour of compulsive eating of certain foods. These are usually refined carbohydrates of the unhealthiest kind, and most children like to drink fizzy pop while eating this 'non-food'.

Hunting dogs in Spain are some of the wildest, most ferocious dogs known. In the weeks before the hunt they are given almost exclusively white bread to eat and water to drink in order to exaggerate their vicious character traits. The dogs lack the nutrients that would be needed to make up for the disease-provoking influence of such unhealthy and unbalanced meals. These highly refined carbohydrates act like a fuse and as soon as the hunt starts and adrenaline is pumped into the system, a chain reaction of chemical substances is set off in the body, increasing the cruelty and speed of these dogs. Their behaviour can be compared to that of hyperactive children who have been eating junk food and drinking sugary drinks for days. When these children are confronted with a stressful situation in the classroom, in a supermarket or at home, they just fly off the handle and cannot control their own behaviour. Sometimes they do not even realise what they are doing and why they are doing it. Their equilibrium has gone and they often feel helpless and totally lost. They do not understand themselves and nobody understands them.

For a long time it has been known that these children may be suffering from a biochemical disorder. A healthy mind requires a regular input of all the right nutrients in the right quantities and proportions, as well as the excretion of as many toxins as possible. Biochemical disorders can sometimes be treated by mega-vitamin therapy and a complete revision of the problematic diet.

❧ *Chapter 9* ❧

DIFFERENT SYMPTOMS

BABIES AND TODDLERS

Although the number of hyperactive or otherwise disturbed children is rising, never make the mistake of classifying your children as hyperactive or different in their behaviour from others unless the symptoms are extremely clear and happen continuously for many weeks or months.

If your child shows some of the symptoms mentioned here, do not worry. Observe your child carefully; although such symptoms can be annoying, you will see that most of them will appear only once in a while and then disappear within a short span of time.

More boys than girls are likely to suffer from hyperactivity. Some symptoms are typical of hyperactivity and similar problems, and others correspond with the behaviour of extremely quiet or autistic children. However, many of the symptoms mentioned in these chapters overlap and can also be seen in normal children once in a while.

A child should not behave like a grown-up person. Children have much more energy than we have and they need to express it all the time. Jumping up and down, running about, racing around or talking non-stop for hours is completely normal. Children can be very naughty or very sweet, because they are going through a period of experimenting and learning. You should accept and understand this. Do not judge and label energetic children or even those who seem to be too quiet. The stigma of such a label could ruin their lives for many years, perhaps forever.

Symptoms that might point towards hyperactivity in infants and young children are:

Crying inconsolably
Difficult feeding
Refuses affection
Does not want to cuddle
Temper tantrums
Screaming and yelling all the time
Head-banging or rocking fits
Restlessness
Aggressiveness (biting and slapping)
Inability to sit still for more than a minute
Destroying own toys and those of other children
Accident-proneness
Bouts of fatigue and weakness
Interrupted sleep
Nose and skin picking and hair pulling
Hypersensitive to lights or sounds
Continuously disobedient
Extreme restlessness
Often fidgeting with hands or feet
Squirming, running, climbing or leaving a seat in situations where quiet behaviour is expected

At the same time there may be physical problems like ear infections, chronic colds, tummy-aches, diarrhoea or constipation, bed-wetting, dark circles or puffiness below the eyes, red earlobes or cheeks, swollen neck glands.

SCHOOL-AGE CHILDREN

School-age children may show some of the same symptoms mentioned above, but besides these there may be:

Quarrelsomeness
Stealing
Resentment of punishments

Clumsiness
Eats junk food or lots of sugar
Likes caffeine (for instance in cola drinks)
Poor muscle coordination
Shows off – a bully
A tendency to hurt others (biting and scratching)
Vandalism
Withdrawn behaviour
Vocal repetition and loudness
Impulsiveness
Disruptive behaviour
Aimless activities
No coordination of movements
School failure
Poor sleep with nightmares
Erratic eating habits
Moodiness or depression
Self-injurious
Hypersensitive to odours, heat and cold
Learning and/or reading disabilities
Unable to complete projects
Unable to make and keep friends
Unable to concentrate

According to the DSM (Diagnostic and Statistical Manual of Mental Disorders), signs of inattention, especially in schoolchildren, include:

Becoming easily distracted by irrelevant sights and sounds
Failing to pay attention to details and making careless mistakes
Rarely following instructions carefully and completely
Blurting out answers before hearing the whole question
Having difficulty waiting in line or for a turn
Losing or forgetting things like toys, or pencils, books and tools needed for a task

In AD/HD, ADD and all similar types of behavioural disorders, hyperactivity is the most prominent characteristic. At the same time there can be poor digestion. It is very important to check the eyesight of these children, as blurred vision and other eye problems may cause some of the symptoms mentioned above.

Many of these children are intelligent, even of above-average intelligence, but they are permanently handicapped by a combination of poor achievement and low self-esteem. Quiet children who are not at all hyperactive but show exactly the opposite personality traits are also often handicapped by their poor achievement and low self-esteem. These children are shy, frightened and love to hide; they often seem to withdraw and disappear within themselves. Sometimes when these symptoms become worse it is called autism, and can be even more dangerous and harder to cure than hyperactivity. Autism can sometimes be detected when the child is still a baby.

Some symptoms are:

Anxiety
Fearfulness
Staying close to their mother
Mood swings
Seeming withdrawn
Daydreaming
Feeling insecure
Skin problems
Unable to communicate
Staying in the corner of a room for hours without playing
Loss of appetite
Clumsiness
Frequent depression
Lethargy

Physical signs can be:

Numbness
Tremors

Blurred vision
Dizziness
Hypoglycaemia (low blood sugar)
Bed-wetting (in older children)

Some patients may show many of these patterns of behaviour. Symptoms overlap and can also be seen in some cases of hyperactivity or the other way around. Atypical behaviour usually appears early in life, before the age of seven, and continues for at least six months.

Again I want to advise you strongly against classifying a quiet and serious child as being mentally retarded or autistic. Each child has its own personality and reacts differently to its environment; to be quiet is for some children completely normal. If you are really worried about the behaviour of your child, first try to find out if your child has any emotional problems he or she cannot cope with. Like grown-ups, there are also children who take real or imagined problems far more to heart than others.

Most of the children that show AD/HD related symptoms will have physical as well as behavioural problems. Usually their intestinal flora is unhealthy. This means that due to bad eating habits or allergic reactions to some foods the bacteria in their intestines are of the wrong kind. As a consequence, even when they begin eating healthily, the nutrients from food they eat cannot be assimilated and used. Cleansing the intestinal tract is very important and it is often amazing how much a child improves after this has been done.

When I was young these problems were hardly known and now they have become one of the most frightening enigmas of our time. All of us should realise that not only the authorities, but every one of us is responsible for this frightening development.

❧ Chapter 10 ❧

POSSIBLE CAUSES

Nobody has ever found a clear connection between AD/HD and family life. Scientists are finding more and more evidence that AD/HD and other behavioural problems stem from biological causes. Some of these disorders can be due to things that happened to the mother during pregnancy: illness, a negative experience or an emotional shock. The nervous system of children can be harmed by medication or drugs their mother has taken. Even a regular habit of drinking coffee, black tea and cola can harm the foetus.

After birth, mental and neurological disorders may have their roots in medical interventions, like too many vaccinations. In many countries different vaccinations are compulsory. However, vaccinations are not always safe or effective. The United States government has paid out over a billion dollars to compensate families who have children who have died or suffered ill effects from a vaccine. That vaccinations are not always effective has been proved by the great number of documented cases of diseases or outbreaks in vaccinated populations.

In many industrial countries there are over 30 vaccinations mandated for use before a child is 16 years old, and a child can have as many as 15 shots in the first six months of life! Only a fraction of the true number of vaccine injuries or deaths is reported or compensated for.

It is not without good reason that fears over and opposition to multiple vaccinations are growing. Although in my opinion vaccination might be advisable if there is a danger of epidemics, or when people travel to foreign countries, where they could catch some tropical disease, I am no friend of routine vaccinations. When I was young, I and almost all my schoolfriends had measles, whooping cough and rubella. It is a known fact that after such illnesses children feel better and are healthier than before. In the course of such diseases the body has the opportunity to excrete many toxins and the immune system becomes stronger. The only kind of vaccination that was mandatory in my time was against smallpox, as in those years that disease was still a danger. Now the risk of normal childhood diseases is terribly exaggerated, and it is interesting to observe that the risk of vaccinations is played down, such vaccinations, in fact, being warmly recommended. I would not dare to speculate about why this is so.

There are four important reasons why one has to look very critically at vaccinations.

> Weak and especially small children are not strong enough to tolerate the great number of vaccinations given.
> Vaccinations impair the immune system and weaken the health of our children, and therefore of the entire population.
> Vaccinations often contain mercury (thimerosal) and other toxic pharmaceuticals.
> The risk of serious injury, disability and death are not explained properly.

Some vaccines contain thimerosal (organic mercury), formaldehyde or other pharmaceutical toxins that are used to prevent bacterial contamination. Most whooping cough, tetanus, influenza, diphtheria, meningitis and other vaccines are still being manufactured with thimerosal, and mercury can build up in the body from each vaccine exposure. In many children suffering from behaviour disorders, like AD/HD, hyperactivity and especially autism, high levels of mercury are found.

The number of vaccinations given is really staggering. Triple vaccines in particular, for example MMR, for mumps, measles and rubella, are a terrible strain. The immune system of a small child cannot cope with such a massive influx of toxins.

Children's defences against all kinds of diseases are much lower than five or six decades ago, when by way of normal childhood illnesses their organism was cleansed of most toxins. Now the general health of our children is appalling.

In my opinion, the irresponsible administration of far too many vaccinations in combination with bad living and eating habits and environmental toxins is one of the most important causes of the frightening increase in behaviour disorders.

ADD has been diagnosed for hundreds of years, but more recently it has become more prevalent due to the increased use of chemicals, pollutants or heavy metal toxicity (such as lead, mercury and cadmium). Each day contaminants from packaging materials or pesticide residues from agricultural or post-harvest use leak into our food. Children are the most vulnerable and unsuspecting victims of chemical agriculture methods. Did you know that some apples and peaches are so contaminated that just two bites are unsafe for children under six? Their small bodies, through food, air and water, are being filled with herbicides and pesticides like Atrazine (the most widely used in the US and rated in the EPA's most toxic category), inordinate doses of antibiotics, unstudied genetically modified foods and hormones from meat and dairy products.

EVERYTHING STARTS WITH THE SOIL

In little more than a century, modern agriculture has managed to destroy what nature built up for millions of years. Most fertile soil has been changed into infertile soil and wastelands where nothing will grow. The remaining soil has been ruined and polluted by millions of tons of dangerous chemicals. In this soil most of the important bacteria have been killed. The vegetables and fruit growing in this soil are lacking in micro-nutrients, therefore our food is also deficient in these. The few nutrients left in our food are usually destroyed by industrial endeavours.

Most of our soil has become a dead substance that can yield only weak and diseased plants which lack the necessary nutrients, hormones and enzymes we and our children need for our health. Animals and humans living on these plants cannot be really healthy, as they lack many of the substances needed for our physical and mental health.

Soft drinks, junk food, industrially refined foods and 'non-food' (potato chips, salty snacks, sweets, pastries, desserts), and too much phosphor in the diet, make our children ill. Alcohol, tobacco, coffee and of course drugs are addictive and unhealthy. All the foods mentioned above are part of the interwoven pattern that threatens our health, as well as the physical, and most importantly, the mental health of our children and of future generations.

WATER

Even if we do not drink water, we use it for cooking. At high temperatures some microbes are killed, but many microbes can stay alive at incredibly high temperatures. Toxic metals are not influenced by heat. Most of our drinking water has been contaminated with very small or larger quantities of chemicals and other toxins from agriculture or waste products from factories.

Most heavy metals and chemicals exist in such small quantities in our food and in our body that they cannot be detected. Many of these toxins are accumulative, however, and will eventually interfere with normal, natural processes. Even if the daily intake of these toxins does not exceed the prescribed quantities, accumulation or interaction with other chemicals in the body can be extremely dangerous. Because of a lack of nutrients, the immune system weakens.

CAUSES OF PHYSICAL AND MENTAL DISEASES

Food additives and indirect food additives
Heavy metals
Polluted air and water
Salicylates
Too much noise
The wrong lighting
Strong medication
Suppression of symptoms
Too little sleep, too little fresh air and too little exercise

&e Chapter 11 &e

WHAT'S WRONG WITH OUR FOOD?

Most of the dangers mentioned in the previous chapters are widely known and therefore it seems reasonable to assume that most women can prevent any health problems that may threaten their children.

However, there are still many dangers we are hardly aware of, because industry, over the course of time, has learned how to hide its manipulations and presents its corrupted and modified food in such a way that it may even look better than the real thing. Also, the endless replays of commercial advertising infiltrate, permeate and seep into our daily life and our subconscious.

We have over 1,000 taste buds in our mouth; these become damaged by the regular use of strong condiments, too much salt and the artificial taste-enhancing properties of modern food. Because of this, many people no longer appreciate the more delicate taste of natural products.

At the beginning of the last century most of the food people ate was still unadulterated and free from toxic chemicals, and eating habits were healthier. Sugar and sweets were still a luxury and in most families meals consisted of simple, wholesome food containing many nutrients which we need in order to stay healthy. And, of course, our lifestyle was completely different too. Now all that has changed. In Europe and the USA we live in a time of abundance never known before. In fact, in our part of the world there is more food available than people need. But are we any healthier because of this? No, quite the contrary! Never before in history have so many people been chronically ill.

The food we eat today no longer contains the nutrients needed for the correct functioning of our digestive system, and therefore most of our physical and mental diseases are caused by and start with metabolic disorders.

In my book *Ten Golden Rules for Good Health* I mention some of the substances used to 'improve' our daily food: artificial colours, anti-oxidising substances, preservatives, emulsifiers, thickeners, gelling agents, taste strengtheners, acid agents and regulators, separating agents, foam-preventing agents, modified starches, artificial sweeteners, dough-raising agents, substances for treating the flour etc. About the dangerous interactions of these substances we know next to nothing.

Our food still contains protein, carbohydrate and fat, but most of these have been modified. Many originally natural foods have been overheated, pressed, cooled, tumbled, frozen or dried and during every one of these procedures vital nutrients have been lost and replaced by countless synthetic vitamins and chemical additives. All refined food undergoes profound changes, but our digestive system has not adjusted to such totally altered food, such as white sugar, white flour and overheated oils.

Our average yearly intake of food additives, in addition to about 115 pounds of sugar and 15 pounds of salt, includes 8.4 pounds of corn syrup, 4.2 pounds of dextrose (glucose), and about 10 pounds out of more than 2,000 different additives. Many processed and packaged foods that are legally marketed and sold contain chemical ingredients, herbicide and pesticide residues, industrial pollutants, artificial (chemical) flavours, artificial (chemical) colours, artificial sweeteners, hormones and hormone metabolites, antibiotics and antibiotic metabolites, preservatives, stabilisers and synthetic or genetically altered ingredients. Our daily food contains thousands of micro-constituents (very small particles) of food preservatives and other additives, naturally occurring vitamins, colours and flavours and contaminants such as liquid plastics, leaked from packaging materials, or pesticide residues from agricultural or post-harvest use.

Whatever television commercials tell you, junk foods and

convenience foods are the most expensive. Those foods with the least nutritional value are often the subject of the most expensive advertising campaigns. 'New' foods are invented all the time and up to 10,000 mostly chemical substances are used in industrial countries to enhance the taste and the appearance of such so-called 'food', and make it more attractive. Fast food and ready-made meals that are absolutely useless for health have become best-sellers. Soup, gravies and sauces which contain nothing but salt, flavourings and other chemical ingredients never deserve to be called natural. We are so used to eating products such as potato chips, crisps and all kinds of sweet and salty snacks that we no longer think of them as harmful. Some foods have been refined so much that the consumer often has no idea what he or she is actually eating. However, most people still hold solid beliefs that their government is adequately protecting them from dangerous or unhealthy products or foods.

Of course, our governments do their best to protect consumers. In Europe and the United States there are many official agencies that define which substances can be used as food additives and decide on the maximum concentrations allowed. All additives must be assessed very carefully for their safety. Each additive that has been investigated is assigned an E number, signifying that it has been approved as safe. That is great – now everybody can relax. Is that right? In fact, even with the help of the newest scientific analytical methods, it is almost impossible to ascertain the toxic level of an additive and what quantity could be harmful to us. Besides this, new additives, or derivations of already known additives, are being used all the time and it is hardly possible for the authorities to keep track of, and control, all of them.

Some laboratories still use animals in order to ascertain the toxic degree of certain substances; others use more sophisticated means. Animals, like humans, are living creatures and it seems logical to use animals for such tests. However, animal testing is sometimes unreliable and has brought about some disastrous results. As chemical additives and drugs are always tested on healthy animals, nobody can foresee what effect they will have in the case of a diseased, adult or a weak child.

Because of the growing political influence of groups that defend the rights of animals and because it is forbidden to use humans for these tests, science has started looking for other methods.

There are two test procedures that can be used to ascertain the toxic levels of additives. One of them is to test additives on living cell material from cultured cells or on bacterial cultures. Another possibility is to find suitable chemicals, which can be used in test solutions. Cells and bacteria from cultures are an intrinsic but very simple part of life, therefore their reactions can never be compared with the reactions that take place in a human body, where every second and even every fraction of a second thousands of actions, reactions and counter-reactions take place. Such tests only have a very limited validity, and the same applies to chemical test substances.

One can hardly judge the quantity of additives a child consumes per day. Nobody seems to know, but it is a fact that most children nowadays often ingest more than double the permissible quantity. Every child reacts differently to toxic substances and although some do not seem to be bothered by the innumerable additives in our food, others react strongly.

Personally, I suspect that in the long run, many of these additives will turn out to be harmful to everybody, even to children and grown-ups who do not seem to show any reaction as yet. When people do not show a reaction to a toxic substance, this does not mean that they are in good health. I will give you an example of what I mean.

Two friends are sitting in a bar drinking a little too much. Next day they meet again and one of them complains about a terrible headache, while the other laughs and says he is feeling fine. In that case, the man who has a headache is the healthy one. His self-defence mechanisms and reactions still function like they should. The same thing happens when people smoke their first cigarette. That first time they become quite ill, then less and less until the body has not been left with enough energy to produce a defensive reaction. This, however, does not mean that toxic substances do not do any harm. On the contrary, these toxins accumulate more and more, usually at the weakest place of the organism, until one day the person in question discovers that he or she is chronically ill or perhaps even has cancer.

I am convinced that one of the main reasons why so many of our children become listless or over-agitated, depressed or aggressive, is the continuous daily influx of infinite small quantities of toxins and their accumulation in their bodies and brains. As a consequence of this, both children and adults suffer from personality changes, depressions, hatred, aggression and a wish to destroy, as can be seen daily on the television newsreel. Therefore we should never underestimate the danger of the chemical deluge that threatens to overpower us.

❧ Chapter 12 ❧

SOFT DRINKS – BEWARE!

Before the First World War, the average annual consumption of carbonated soft drinks in the United States was about sixty 12-ounce servings per person. At that time official health professionals of the American Medical Association (AMA) stated: 'From a health point of view it is desirable to have restriction of such use of sugar as is represented by consumption of sweetened carbonated beverages and forms of candy which are of low nutritional value.' They said also that it would be in the interest of public health to limit consumption of sugar in any form in which it failed to be combined with significant proportions of other foods of high nutritive quality. The idea was that soft sugary drinks should only be drunk as an accompaniment to healthy, natural food that contained enough valuable nutrients to compensate for the loss of minerals that results from the consumption of these drinks.

By 2001 the consumption of soft drinks had increased by about ten-fold and provides now at least one-third of all refined sugar in the diet. However, for some reason the AMA and other similar organisations are now largely silent on the subject. Children start drinking pop at a remarkably young age, and consumption increases through young adulthood. One-fifth of one- and two-year-old children consume soft drinks! Those toddlers drink an average of nearly one cup per day.

Carbonated drinks are the single biggest source of refined sugar in the American diet. Teens especially often meet their recommended sugar limits from soft drinks alone. With candy, cookies, cake, ice cream and other sugary foods, most exceed the general recommendations by a large margin and in Europe the situation is not much better. Soft drinks are the fifth-largest source of calories for adults. They pose health risks both because of what they contain (for example, sugar and additives) and what they replace in the diet (foods that provide vitamins, minerals and other nutrients).

Obesity increases the risk of diabetes and cardiovascular disease and causes severe social and psychological problems in millions of people. In the last 30 years, obesity rates in teenagers soared from about 5 per cent to about 14 per cent. At the same time, among adults the rate of obesity jumped from 25 per cent to about 37 per cent.

Numerous factors contribute to obesity. Soft drinks add unnecessary, non-nutritious calories to the diet. Obesity rates have risen in tandem with soft-drink consumption, and heavy consumers of these beverages have higher calorie intakes. National institutes of health in many countries recommend that people who are trying to lose weight should drink water instead of soft drinks with sugar.

TOOTH DECAY (DENTAL CARIES)

Refined sugar is one of several important factors that promote tooth decay. A regular intake of soft drinks promotes tooth decay because these drinks bathe the teeth in sugary water for long periods of time during the day. To prevent tooth decay, even the Canadian Soft Drink Association recommends limiting between-meal snacking on sugary and starchy foods, avoiding prolonged sugar levels in the mouth, eating sugary foods and drinking sugary beverages with meals. Unfortunately, most heavy drinkers of soft drinks violate each of those precepts.

Several additives in soft drinks raise health concerns. Caffeine, a mildly addictive stimulant drug, is present in most cola and 'pepper' drinks, as well as in some orange sodas and other products. Caffeine addiction may be one reason why six of the seven most popular soft drinks contain caffeine. Coca-Cola and other companies have begun marketing soft drinks such as Surge, Josta and Jolt, which contain 30–60 per cent more caffeine than Coke and Pepsi.

One problem with caffeine is that it increases the excretion of calcium in the urine. Caffeine can also cause nervousness, irritability, sleeplessness and a rapid heartbeat. It causes children to be restless and fidgety, develop headaches and have difficulty going to sleep. Caffeine addiction may keep people hooked on soft drinks (or other caffeine-containing beverages). Several additives used in soft drinks cause occasional allergic reactions. Yellow 5 dye causes asthma, hives and a runny nose. Natural red colourings, like cochineal and carmine, can cause life-threatening reactions. Dyes can cause hyperactivity in sensitive children.

Soft-drink companies are among the most aggressive marketeers in the world. Their advertising budgets dwarf all advertising and public-service campaigns promoting the consumption of fruit and vegetables, and a healthy lifestyle. Between 1986 and 1997 soft-drink companies spent 6.8 billion dollars on advertising. Americans and also many Europeans have come to consider soft drinks a routine snack and a standard, appropriate part of meals instead of an occasional treat. Moreover, many of today's younger parents grew up with soft drinks themselves and see their routine consumption as normal, so they make little effort to restrict their children's consumption of them. Soft drinks may contribute to dental problems, kidney stones and heart disease. The additives in them may cause insomnia, behavioural problems and allergic reactions.

The industry promises that it will do everything possible to persuade still more people to drink even more soft drinks, more often. Parents and health officials need to recognise soft drinks for what they are – liquid candy – and do everything possible to return those beverages to their former, reasonable role as an occasional treat.

In the UK 1,000 glasses of soft drinks are drunk every second. This is a per capita consumption of 186 litres per annum. In the rest of Europe this is 202 litres and in the USA 400 litres. With children drinking nearly 200 litres of soft drinks per head in the UK alone, soft drink manufacturers are increasingly focusing their marketing efforts on the younger generation. Consumption of soft drinks by children under five has doubled over the past 15 years, and doctors warn that this could lead to a generation of malnourished youngsters. The problem is that there are children drinking up to three pints of calorie-laden soft drinks every day, which is destroying their appetites and can lead to a nutrient deficiency in their diets.

A study at Southhampton General Hospital found that 15 per cent of two- to four-year-olds were getting nearly half their recommended energy intake from soft drinks.

These findings are even more worrying in the light of a survey released at the same time that revealed two out of three children are eating such a poor diet that they fail to meet the government's minimal nutritional guidelines. The survey also discovered an alarming ignorance among mothers about what constitutes a healthy diet.

❧ Chapter 13 ❧

SUGAR

When we were small my brother used to love any kind of sweets, pastry, chocolate or sweet-tasting drinks. I remember that he was always chewing or nibbling at something and if he did not get something sweet, he became quite nasty. My mother said that even as a baby he had a 'sweet tooth', and she usually gave in to him when he started crying or yelling in order to get what he wanted. When we grew up, he spent most of his pocket money on sweets, pastries and anything else made of white flour and sugar, as well as on soft drinks. Every year he gained more weight; he did not like sports and most of the time he sat in front of the television watching his favourite programmes.

When he was 15 years old, the doctor told him that if he did not live more healthily he would soon become a diabetic. Diabetes ran in the family and one of our uncles was in a wheelchair because of the disease. Years ago his toes had started to turn blue and later black, and they had to amputate one of his feet. When my brother heard what the doctor had said, he began to panic. Then our uncle told him that his own poor health was due to his sweet tooth when he was a child, and he decided there and then to stop eating sweets.

We did really not believe that he could do it, but to our great surprise, my brother had enough willpower to get over his addiction. In the beginning it was awfully hard for him, but always in his mind he saw the stump of his uncle's leg and this gave him the courage to fight on. In order to suppress his cravings, he often ate some fruit or raw vegetables, like carrots or fennel, and after some time they stopped. After a couple of years his blood sugar had become normal again, and he lost weight and started doing sports. Now he is a healthy man, happily married with a lovely wife and two children. He has not become a fanatic, but he and his family love to eat wholesome and simple food.

How does such a craving for sweets start, and why is it that some people have this problem and others do not? In order to understand this we have to go back about 200 years. At that time no refined foods and few sweets of any kind were available and diseases like diabetes were hardly known. Sugar existed, but it was very expensive. There was even a time when people kept their sugar in a special 'sugar box', that only could be opened with a special key! (How wonderful it would be and how much disease could be prevented if one could reinstall this custom today.)

In our time everyone can afford to buy cheap, refined sugar, which is totally different from the natural substance found, for example, in fruit. Through extraction, heating, bleaching etc., the manufacturers have produced an artificial concentrated product which contains hardly any nutrients, only calories. Sugar has been turned into a lifeless substance that endangers our health if consumed regularly. This applies to any kind of sugar, perhaps with the exception of *small quantities* of unadulterated natural honey or cane sugar.

In the process of extraction from the sugar cane or beet, all fibre, vitamins, minerals and other nutrients that are present in the plant are discarded. The biggest problem is that the human organism cannot metabolise sugar or any other refined food when the original nutrients are missing. As soon as these refined products are eaten, a message goes from the sensible taste buds and nerves in the mouth to the brain with a demand for the nutrients that are needed in order to metabolise this refined food. The brain reacts by taking vitamins and minerals from its reserves in the bones, from the muscles and above all from the nervous system, at the same time sending a message to the pancreas to release more insulin. All this happens because in nature, sugar is always a component part, for example of a fruit. Sugar is always combined with fibre, and with all the nutrients needed for the breaking up, assimilation and utilisation of the entire fruit. When eating a fruit, root or vegetable, the pancreas will always make the exact amount of insulin that is needed for the assimilation of these foods and the blood sugar stays constant. However, when pure refined sugar enters our mouth, the pancreas does not change its former habits and still releases all the insulin needed for the digestion of the entire fruit this sugar originally came from. Of course in that case there will be a big surplus of insulin that is not needed for the digestion of the small quantity of concentrated sugar and all the digestive processes turn topsy-turvy.

When that happens we feel a craving for something sweet and our blood sugar level drops lower and lower. This condition is called hypoglycaemia; it not only may cause extreme weakness, dizziness or even circulatory diseases, but is also one of the most important causes of hyperactivity and some other personality changes in children. Many children are addicted to sweets and other non-foods or soft drinks, and they feel better only when they eat something that normalises their blood sugar for a short time.

Sugar is not a poison, but it becomes a big problem when used regularly in large quantities. The situation becomes even worse when sugar is combined with other kinds of 'refined' foods. Then the body will be depleted of many essential nutrients. Refined foods, especially sugar, rob the nervous system of B vitamins and other nutrients. Without these nutrients our nerves and our brain cannot function normally. No wonder that kids who consume large quantities of junk food and sugary drinks often behave strangely, become aggressive and restless, and show in 100 different ways that something is wrong with them.

Food manufacturers love to use sugar. In the first place sugar is one of the best preservatives for all kinds of food. Bacteria cannot live in such a highly concentrated substance; but this also means that the good bacteria in our intestines, needed for the processing of our food, cannot stay healthy when we eat refined food regularly. Secondly, manufacturers love to use sugar because it is addictive, and everything prepared with it sells extremely well. In the third place sugar can disguise the bad taste and spoilage of certain products.

The market has been inundated with sugar and other refined foods and drinks and our children are the victims of our careless attitude and business manipulations. Even in or near our schools, children are tempted to spend their pocket money on sugary snacks and drinks.

Some children are so sensitive to sugar that anything that contains the smallest amount of it makes them go almost crazy. Some studies disagree with this. However, as we know that sugar is never healthy for anybody, it would be advisable to use it as little as possible anyway.

It is usually extremely difficult to keep children away from sugar. However, there are several natural sweeteners that can be used instead, like organic brown rice syrup, barley malt, wild agave syrup, natural maple syrup, liquorice and others.

The best and most natural sweetener is stevia. This is a sweet herb that has been used for thousands of years by people in Paraguay, South America. Stevia is used in Japan to make coca drinks sweet. One can try to buy and grow this little plant at home, although it is not easy to get hold of. To use stevia leaf, simply make a tea (half a teaspoon to a cup of water, let steep for 15 minutes). In some countries stevia is available commercially as drops, powder or dried leaves. One should use very little stevia, as it is so sweet that if you use just a little too much the taste becomes bitter. One or two drops in a cup of herbal tea are sufficient. It is understandable that the FDA and some governmental institutions in other countries are trying to prevent the importation and sale of this herb, as they want to support the sugar industry. Wonderful herb teas, like chamomile, peppermint, spearmint, orange peel, cinnamon and hibiscus sweetened with stevia or liquorice taste very good indeed. Children should drink them instead of harmful soft drinks.

❧ Chapter 14 ❧

LOW BLOOD SUGAR

Many physical and mental problems are caused by low blood sugar (hypoglycaemia). This is a disturbance in the metabolism of sugar. Low blood sugar is a widespread condition, even in the smallest of children, and often goes unrecognised. A child could be categorised as listless, with no interest in school, or easily distracted and unable to maintain concentration on a subject, when his or her brain is incapable of functioning properly due to insufficient fuel.

Some well-meaning parents are still under the impression that sugar, any kind of sugar, is good for the brain. 'The brain needs sugar, and my child eats a good deal of sugar,' a loving parent might say. But that is exactly the problem. What the brain needs continually, besides oxygen, is glucose, not sucrose. After consuming food or beverages containing industrial sugar, i.e. sucrose in an isolated form, the blood sugar will soar within minutes. Then the pancreas will supply insulin, needed for the digestion of this sugar. Soon the job will be done; the sugar will be digested and usually after one or two hours or even sooner, the blood sugar level falls far below normal. This triggers an immediate craving for more candy and soft drinks, and a chain reaction will follow. Frequent consumption of food or beverages containing refined sugar can easily induce low blood sugar (hypoglycaemia) as an almost constant condition. As a consequence of a chronic low blood sugar the normal functions of the pancreas are disturbed. Because of this, hypoglycaemia is often a preliminary stage of hyperglycaemia (high blood sugar) and diabetes, which lately has been increasing at a frightening speed all over the world. If people with these conditions do not change their eating and drinking habits, they will suffer for it. Some starchy foods, like wholegrain cereals, will maintain a steady level of blood sugar, whereas starches like white bread, white rice, white noodles etc. can also be responsible for excessive variations of the blood sugar level, although not as extreme as refined sugar.

Many children eat hardly anything for breakfast and when they do eat something, it usually does them more harm than good. These children and most parents do not have the slightest idea of what they should eat and what is healthy. A meal of chocolate milk and a doughnut contains much refined sugar, refined flour and plenty of phosphorus and other additives. The sugar is digested in no time, the blood sugar goes up and energy is produced. So far, so good.

The child leaves for school and feels fine. However, the energy that came from his breakfast will be spent very soon and in one or two hours at the most all the energy from his breakfast has been used up. At the same time the phosphorus in the milk depletes the organism and the nervous system of much-needed calcium.

Many children spend too much time indoors, and therefore have a lack of sunshine and light and consequently of vitamin D. Vitamin D is needed for the absorption of calcium. The best source of vitamin D is cod-liver oil, which our grandparents took by the spoonful. Modern children, even if they do not suffer from hyperactivity and similar problems, may become nervous and excited, and have sleeping problems because of a lack of calcium and other essential nutrients. It is possible to get enough calcium from vegetables, nuts and other natural foods, but many children hardly ever eat these and their parents do not give the right example; even doctors usually know far too little about food.

Let me return to children who become hungry while at school. As a snack, they prefer to eat something sweet. They are very tired, but they know that as soon as they eat or drink something sweet their energy comes right back. However, this new energy behaves in the same way as the energy that was produced during breakfast and will be used up in a very short time. At the end of the morning these children are half asleep and often do not even realise what the teacher is saying.

A continuous drop in blood sugar causes fatigue to become exhaustion. Children may suffer from headaches and weakness and their little brains cannot function well because the brain needs the right kind of sugar. Even when the amount of sugar in the blood falls just a little below normal, not only children but also grown-ups become irritable, moody and uncooperative.

If children start the day with the right kind of breakfast, they will have plenty of energy until lunch. What is the right kind of breakfast? Certainly not chocolate milk and a sugary doughnut. Try to find something healthy that the child still enjoys. Although children all have their own personal likes and dislikes, there are some general rules. The first is that children should enjoy their food. Children who do not like what they are eating will have a bad digestion and their health will deteriorate. Never force children to eat something they do not like.

The second rule is not to let your child get into the habit of eating between meals. If they do, it should certainly not be crisps or sweets, and never soft drinks. Of course they should not have those during mealtimes either! If your child is really hungry between meals, you can provide some raisins, nuts or an apple, but never too much. If children's tummies are not empty at mealtimes, they have no appetite and will not eat the nutritious food that provides all the fuel that the body and brain need.

Do not treat children who are older than about five as if they are babies. Explain to them they will not be able to run and play so well if they eat the wrong things, and when they get a bit older that their skin may be ruined and they will not look as good if they have lots of junk food and soft drinks. Talk with your children as friends and answer their questions. If you yourself do not know some of the answers, buy books about health and study them well instead of giving the wrong answers. Your children have to trust you and they should know that their parents are right.

If your child already suffers from hyperactivity or another behavioural problem, always remember that hyperactive children do not do it on purpose; they do not destroy things or behave badly deliberately. They are victims of an imbalance in their bodies and minds, and most of the time this is due to toxins, wrong eating habits and other causes. Many of these causes are reversible and you should explain this to your child. Most children are far more intelligent than we realise, and because they have not yet learned the wrong things we were taught, they understand in some respects even more than we do. While lecturing to families or talking to my grandchildren I often notice this.

Do not change bad habits straightaway; go slowly and carefully. Always let your child know what you are doing and why you are doing it. Children love to be treated like grown-ups and to participate, especially when they discover that they feel better when they are not eating crisps or sweets, or drinking soft drinks. After some time their bodies will become used to the right kind of food and they will start liking it and be proud to be able to do something about their own problems.

For breakfast you could serve different herb teas and let them choose which of three or four kinds they like best. You can add a little lemon and maybe some natural honey, but at first try to let your child taste it without adding anything sweet. If it is not sweet enough add a few drops of stevia (the wonderful natural sweetener from South America). Wholewheat crackers or rolls with butter, and a soft boiled egg with a little herbal salt, or boiled porridge with a little honey, natural maple syrup or dried fruit all make a good breakfast. If you serve porridge, add some almonds or nuts; children need protein every morning with breakfast. It allows the blood sugar to go up slowly and will provide energy for many hours.

Do not give your child anything with sugar or with refined flour to take to school. Nuts, raisins and other dried or fresh fruit, like an apple or a pear, make the best snacks. A nice cucumber sandwich on wholewheat bread is a more substantial but very healthy snack. However, children should be feeling hungry again by lunchtime.

For lunch you could prepare a lovely salad, varying the type each day, from different raw vegetables or lettuce. Never buy commercial salad dressings, as they are full of preservatives and other bad things. You can make an excellent salad dressing at home with cold-pressed oil, a little lemon or wine vinegar, different herbs, and a little herbal salt or sea-salt. Taste it; it should not be too sour. Home-made mayonnaise, diluted with very little water, also makes a nice dressing.

For cooked vegetable dishes, steam the vegetables without any fat or butter. When you dish these up, you can put some butter or cold-pressed oil on them and add a little herbal salt. Or put the dish in the oven for a short time with some grated cheese and butter. If your child is allergic to milk, replace the cheese with breadcrumbs and a little butter. You can make a nice potato salad with some chopped-up onions, a little vinegar and herb salt, as well as some kitchen herbs. Let your children help in the kitchen – they will enjoy doing this. Maybe after some time they themselves might come up with some new ideas.

Twice a week you could prepare some fish and once or twice a week some meat. Experiment with different ways of cooking it to find out what your child likes. Instead of a high tea with biscuits and cakes, give your child wholemeal radish or lettuce sandwiches with butter or mayonnaise.

Most of the things you buy should be fresh and wholesome and if you exceptionally buy tinned food like sardines or tuna fish, read the ingredients very carefully and never buy anything that has E numbers listed. After your children have eaten simple and wholesome food, and no junk food, for a few weeks, you will be amazed at how much they have changed for the better. With wholesome food the blood sugar rises slowly and energy will be available for many hours. Your children will be less tired and after some time their behaviour will improve. This is no fairytale; it has been proved many times over.

A child whose diet is faulty usually suffers from multiple and overlapping deficiencies. Children who suffer from hyperactivity and other mental and emotional problems often have two things in common: low blood sugar and an over-sensitivity to phosphorus.

This is not a cookbook, so I have only given you a general idea of what you could make. You love your children and you really can help them, so please try. You will be amazed at the results; the best thing is that a child who has suffered from low blood sugar can have a completely normal blood sugar level and will feel so much better. Hypoglycaemia is a condition brought on by a protein-poor, vitamin-poor, high-carbohydrate diet.

❧ Chapter 15 ❧

FOOD ALLERGIES AND
INCOMPATIBILITIES

Formerly infections were the most frequent causes of disease. In our time allergies, mainly caused by food, are increasing uncontrollably. Over 70 per cent of the population of industrial countries has an allergic disposition. When speaking of an allergy, we mean a changed or unusual defensive reaction against some well-known, or unknown, substance. An allergic disposition can be hereditary or acquired. An allergic reaction to a substance or food can happen within seconds or over a period of up to 72 hours. Innumerable health problems or even serious illness can be caused by allergens. Most affected are the skin and the mucous membranes.

There is no need to describe the very complicated process that can trigger off an allergic reaction. This subject has often been discussed. However, what we want to know is *why* we actually become allergic. Usually people become allergic because for some reason their liver is unable to detoxify the offending substances. This is often due to an overload of toxins.

Until about 100 years ago an allergy was something out of the ordinary. Now it is officially accepted that the contamination of our modern environment has created a climate propitious for the development of such illnesses. We can get an allergy at any time in life, even as a bottle-fed baby. The digestive system of the baby was designed to deal with its mother's milk, which has a completely different quality and composition from cows' milk. The digestion of the foreign protein in cows' milk is far from easy for a baby and the great surplus of phosphorus and other factors is also problematic.

An allergic reaction to cows' milk is the dominant problem during the first year of life. Often the organism excretes the offending substances by way of the skin and therefore many babies get skin problems, for example the so-called 'milk crust'. If these skin problems are suppressed by medication or creams, more serious diseases may develop and the baby may retain an allergic disposition throughout its entire life. Such a baby will be very sensitive to all kinds of allergens, not only to those from milk and milk products. Allergic reactions in infancy are expressed as crying, colic, excessive vomiting, diarrhoea, rashes, eczema and cold-like respiratory congestion.

Both industrial and natural products can contain allergens (substances which trigger off allergic reactions in the body) from agriculture or cattle breeding. One can have an allergic reaction to almost anything, and such a reaction can take place in any part of the body. An allergic disposition can lie dormant for many years and break out only after someone comes into contact with certain substances while the defensive forces are under par.

Children who suffer from bronchitis, sinusitis or asthma often owe their condition to an allergic disposition. When the cause of the allergy is discovered and removed, it is often surprising how quickly many health problems disappear, but most of the time it is very difficult to isolate allergens.

The most common problems are sore throats, ear infections, lymphnode swelling, digestive disorders, skin eruptions, especially eczema and hives, respiratory problems (from a runny nose to asthma and pneumonia), headaches, muscle and joint pains, and abdominal pain. Usually there are mental disturbances at the same time. The earliest mental disturbances to manifest themselves are irritability, moodiness and sleep disorders, especially nightmares and night terrors. Some children are hyperactive and difficult to manage. Other children wilt and withdraw (autism).

An allergic reaction may be against: milk or other dairy products, refined cane sugar, industrial cocoa, chocolate, corn, eggs, wheat, soy, citrus fruits, monosodium glutamate, preservatives, dyes, caffeine, sweeteners, saturated fats, pork, eggs, strong cheese, margarine, cornflakes, peanuts, Brazil nuts, coffee, nicotine, Brussels sprouts, artichokes, savoy cabbage, peas and hundreds of other things. Vegetables from the nightshade family, like tomatoes, aubergines and potatoes, can also be food allergens.

The body tries to defend itself against allergens in different ways and when one defensive measure is exhausted, it will try another. This situation can be compared to an army. When troops are unable to continue to fight, other units take over. Maybe the next battle will then be fought somewhere else with different weapons. In our body, first there will be a reaction that takes place by way of the skin. Later these reactions may take place deeper in the body; far more diseases are caused by allergens – that is, by substances our body cannot cope with – than we generally believe.

Unfortunately, most doctors know hardly anything about allergies and treat, for example, asthma or bronchitis with medication that suppresses the symptoms. That the patient in question could be allergic to cows' milk, sugar, chocolate, beer or certain chemical substances in the food is completely ignored. Because of ignorance, millions of patients have to take suppressive medication for their whole lives. Those with chronic health problems should try to cut out of their diets, for at least one or two weeks, any food they eat regularly. It is very possible that a health problem a patient has had for years will disappear completely when the offensive substance is taken away.

People who get allergic reactions after eating their favourite food should refrain from having it in the future. Allergic problems can also be traced by watching a change in behaviour patterns. There can be allergic reactions to ordinary foods, but also to substances we come into contact with everyday, like cleaning fluids, aerosols or petrol fumes.

THE ALLERGY RIDDLE

According to some physicians, hyperactivity and behavioural problems have nothing to do with allergic reactions. That, of course, is a matter of opinion. It is undeniable that there are usually not one, but several (often overlapping) causes. The meaning of the word 'allergy' has been defined differently through the ages and the most recent explanations of allergic reactions are so complicated that only a few specialised physicians may find their way through the maze.

About 100 years ago hardly anybody would have thought that mental diseases, physical problems or unusual behaviour could have anything to do with a reaction to certain foods, or substances in these foods. This changed when some doctors in North America, Britain and later Germany started to look into these problems. Scientists like Ted Randolph, Herbert Rinkel, Albert Rowe, George Watson, Professor Comrey, Richard Mackarness, Professor Pfister, Lothar Burgerstein, Anna Calantin and many others achieved outstanding results by treating food allergies. Their achievements were so amazing that we should never overlook them. In his clinic near London, Richard Mackarness treated and cured uncountable allergic patients. It also became known that Hippocrates, in 460 BC, and other famous doctors of antiquity were convinced that mental diseases and abnormal behaviour were often caused by a malfunction of the metabolism and not by a sick mind or a bad or unbalanced personality. Even in those early times patients improved when their eating habits were changed and they were treated with laxatives and emetics.

Knowing all this, we are able to draw some conclusions. Firstly, long ago some abnormal diseases were caused by the wrong metabolic reactions, and this means that some people, even in those times, could not metabolise (digest) certain foods. Of course, in 460 BC food additives and chemical pollution of the environment were non-existent, but it is exactly these that are mainly responsible for the overwhelming increase of behavioural problems and mental diseases of our time.

In Hippocratic times most food was still natural. However, people soon realised that oil- or fat-containing food did not taste good after a while, as it became rancid. Therefore the first food that was heated intensively must have been oil. Today oil is still an enigmatic problem. Rancid oil is uneatable and dangerous for our health. However, when oil has been exposed to high temperatures, it becomes 'saturated' and loses its healthy qualities. Cold-pressed oil, extracted during the first pressing of olives or other oleaginous (oil-containing) fruit or vegetables, still becomes rancid if the rules to prevent this are not observed. Bottles should be hermetically sealed and should be stored in a dark place, as light can spoil this very sensitive oil. All manufacturers of industrially heated oils fear rancidity, and therefore add several additives to oil, butter and other fatty and perishable food. The dangers of these additives are explained later on.

It is quite possible that in olden times people were not allergic to the foods themselves, but to the rancid fats in the food. Milk also soon becomes spoiled and rancid when unheated. In the past many newborn babies died when their mothers were unable to feed them and they were given animal milk. This had much to do with the unhygienic conditions in which the milk was kept in those times. Today these problems have increased many times over, as most foods children like, even if they are able to metabolise the food itself, contain additives and other toxic substances. It is almost impossible to find food that is not contaminated in this way. Even 'natural' fruit and vegetables come from a soil that is full of chemicals and lacks the most important nutrients. Most fruit and vegetables are sprayed and packed into plastic or other wrappings or containers made from artificial and toxic materials, which can leak into the food.

We should not forget that the body needs a lot of energy in order to fight against the flood of dangerous chemicals we face in modern life. This energy is badly needed for defence against disease and other important tasks. It is extremely important to find out what kind of foods or substances your child is sensitive or allergic to, so that you can omit them and at least try to prevent this loss of energy.

More and more people are allergic to milk and dairy products. Different kinds of cereals, especially wheat, refined carbohydrates, eggs, citrus fruits (mainly when they have been sprayed or waxed), tomatoes, tinned food, chocolate, sausages, pork and breakfast cereals cause similar reactions. If you suspect that your child might be allergic to a food he eats quite often, you should cut it out completely from his diet for four to five days, and then try a little of this food, no more than a teaspoon on the child's empty stomach in the morning. If there is a negative reaction, like a headache, a rapid heartbeat, vomiting or other signs of feeling unwell, it is a sign that in future you should no longer give your child that particular food. In this way you can test many different kinds of food, and find out which of them causes a reaction. In some hospitals and clinics which specialise in food allergies or similar problems, the same kind of method is used.

However, testing at home also has its advantages and often the results of such tests can help you and your child very much indeed. In my clinic, patients often are put on a so-called water-fast for a few days. During this time they are not allowed to eat anything; they drink only water, so that their digestive tract becomes as clean as possible. After that the testing begins.

FOOD INTOLERANCES

Preschool infants with food problems tend to become fussy or picky eaters with strong food preferences and refuse to eat many healthy foods. Children with food allergies typically become eating specialists, compulsively eating a small number of favourite foods and refusing the rest. Vegetable foods are often the first foods refused.

Food allergies are quite easy to detect, but it is far more difficult to detect intolerance to a certain food. The symptoms can become evident up to 30 hours or more after the questioned ingredient has been introduced. In the case of hyperactivity or difficulty in prolonged concentration, food intolerance should be a suspect. Experts say that at least one in every two children suffers from intolerance to one or more food substances.

The blood test for allergies does not reveal this problem. There may be an extreme addiction to a particular food or drink. Children may become irritable or impatient if they cannot have it. The same thing happens when a drug addict stops taking drugs; the 'drug effect' is the symptom of withdrawal crisis!

❧ Chapter 16 ❧

THE PHOSPHORUS CONNECTION

Besides a genetic predisposition, nutrition is the most important factor for the development of a human being and in that area too much phosphorus in the daily food can have serious consequences.

Phosphorus is one of the essential components of our nutrition. There is very little possibility of a deficiency, since today most people consume far too much of it. Between 1940 and 2001 our daily intake of phosphorus went from 800 mg to an average of about 1,600 mg daily. This is twice the recommended daily intake of 800 mg for people of 25 and over, and 1,200 mg for young people from 11–24 years and pregnant women.

Our organism is unprepared for the assimilation of such great quantities of one specific kind of food component. We do not know yet what side-effects there may be in the long run, but children especially and teenagers, who certainly have a lion's share of the new food fads, might be risking mild or even severe toxic reactions.

Few people realise that our organism reacts in a very sensitive manner to an overload of phosphorus. Some of us who have had the opportunity to learn something about biological agriculture know that by putting too much phosphorus and other things into the soil, the soil becomes over-saturated. Such soil cannot assimilate other elements, which in much smaller quantities are often at least as important for the health of the soil and the plants growing in it. On this planet everything functions according to the same laws and rules, so it could easily be possible that what happens in the soil may also happen in the human body. If our organism contains too much phosphorus and the body has become saturated with it, the assimilation of other, much-needed nutrients might become impossible. If the influx of phosphorus continues and the body cannot be freed from the overload, within a short time there will be a serious lack of other, still more important nutrients and this may have disastrous consequences.

The first reaction occurs when babies are given cows' milk formulas for the first time. Cows' milk has a different composition and contains almost six times as much phosphorus as mothers' milk. Only a few babies are able to assimilate such a quantity. They often react with milk crust or croup and this can signal the onset of all kinds of allergies. Proneness to phosphorous sensitivity is passed on as a hereditary characteristic of the metabolism and may be one of the most important causes of behavioural disorders.

Phosphorus and calcium should be present proportionately in a ratio of about 50/50, but in modern food there is usually far more phosphorus than calcium because of the huge amounts our soil now contains. Too much phosphorus inhibits the assimilation of calcium. The more phosphorus there is, the less calcium will be available and as our modern food contains far less calcium than the food our grandparents ate anyway, this is a very serious problem. Excess phosphorus combines with minerals, forming insoluble salts in the intestines and urinary tract. When these are excreted, not only calcium but a great deal of important minerals are lost.

A lack of vitamin D, sunlight and other factors also plays a role in these processes and we know that one of the consequences of too little calcium is brittle bones. Too much phosphorus causes acidity and this acid has to be neutralised by calcium. If there is not enough calcium intake with the daily food, it will be taken out of the bones and the teeth. However, this is not the only purpose of calcium. Calcium is needed not only for physical, but also for mental processes. As well as other functions, calcium plays a role in cell division and the transmission of neural impulses. Adults need about 1 gram of calcium a day, but nowadays even that quantity is seldom reached in our industrial countries.

Scientists have found that after only one meal containing phosphorus additives, calcium was mobilised out of the bones.

Furthermore, and this is very important concerning the health problems discussed in this book, calcium helps control the acid–alkali balance of our blood. The metabolism of many children suffering from hyperactivity and mental problems is very alkaline. This can be measured by checking the alkaline level of the saliva, which should be done first thing in the morning. At night, instead of giving your restless child medication with dangerous side-effects, you could give him or her half a teaspoon of pure wine vinegar in a cup of water and see what happens. As the alkali will now be replaced by acid, you may be in for a happy surprise. It would be worthwhile to give this a try.

If your child does not show a positive reaction to the vinegar, leave it, but if there is a positive reaction by all means continue with the treatment. Your child may become more quiet and relaxed as a result. You can repeat this a few times a day and especially at night-time, because vinegar will help your child to sleep better, but do not increase the quantity. Vinegar has been part of our nutrition for thousands of years and it can do no harm. However, do not give too much at a time, as too much of a good thing is always bad. Many children seem to like the taste of vinegar; maybe this is a natural response to their need for some acidity once in a while. Vinegar helps, but citric acid, malic acid (from apples) or other kinds of acids do not.

More boys than girls are sensitive to phosphorus. For most of their lives women are more or less protected against some of the negative influences in their diet because of their feminine hormones (oestrogen), even when they are still children. After the menopause this protection disappears and from that time on, phosphorus can endanger their calcium metabolism. If they knew more about nutrition there would be nothing to fear. Testosterone (the male hormone), on the other hand, offers no defence against the harmful effects of too much phosphorus in the diet.

Children who have a strong reaction to anything containing phosphorus can often be helped by a phosphorus-free diet. Some children, after eating such a diet for at least four days, may change completely; others need about two weeks. You may have to experiment, but do not lose faith.

❧ Chapter 17 ❧

FOOD ADDITIVES

First, let us hear what the food industry once had to say about food additives.

Forty years ago an interesting press release by a spokesman of the food industry appeared in the media. It read:

> Most people are not yet able to appreciate all the considerable benefits of food additives. The greatest benefits stem primarily from the role of these chemicals in increasing food production, in conserving foods in storage, and in making food continuously available. Unbelievable quantities of perishable, spoiling food could be saved and given to the needy people of this world. Always new and better additives might within some decades fulfil our dream of a world without hunger. The benefits greatly outweigh any hazard detected by present methods of toxicology and safety evaluation.

Although 40 years ago many people still believed in the magic of antibiotics and other wonder drugs, even most physicians are not so sure any more that antibiotics are a panacea for every ill. People now are coming to realise more and more the unforeseeable dangers involved in the use of hitherto unknown chemicals. Sometimes it is only after many decades that their devastating properties are discovered. By then it is usually far too late to prevent terrible suffering or early death.

Now we recognise that there could be real dangers connected with the use of all those once celebrated chemical preservatives, colourings, taste-enhancers and similar products. We realise that scientific studies and laboratory tests can never give us the proof of absolute safety. Scientifically, long-term hazards can never be demonstrated, for example what would happen if these chemicals were ingested by small children, or weak and diseased people.

The public is anxious and does not accept the explanations of the food industry any more. The change in children's behaviour, bad manners, bad moods, nervousness, hyperactivity, aggressiveness, criminal conduct and even autism cannot be solely the consequence of bad parenting and a lack of love or education. There is something definitely wrong with our children and teenagers and in some respects even with ourselves.

Is it too far-fetched to look for chemical culprits invading our brain and nerve cells when the normal reactions and behaviour of so many people are changing? Why do people believe that it is only the personalities of drug addicts or patients with mental health problems that change when they are taking chemical medication? Chemicals, or even natural substances, can provoke reactions in the human body in dilutions of a thousand or even a million to one. We can smell flowers or rubbish from far away, and that means that part of our brain reacts to unbelievably high dilutions.

It is very possible that when natural foods are changed in a drastic way and all kinds of chemical substances added, our organism reacts and crucial changes take place in our personality. Pregnant women, babies and young children are very sensitive to chemical substances in high dilutions. It does not mean anything that such changes cannot yet be proved by the usual scientific methods. At the present time, food additives are not yet being tested for behavioural or developmental changes.

Already quite a few experts agree that a lifetime of ingesting such chemicals could play a major role in causing birth defects, cancer, chemical sensitivity, decreased immune function, degenerative health conditions, food allergies and nerve damage. It is quite possible that the human race is in greater danger from a general chemical flooding than from atomic warfare.

Consumer safety is very important, especially regarding food additives. To protect consumers, food legislation in the European Union and in the United States defines which substances can be used as food additives. In most cases such legislation also lists the foods in which each additive can be used and the maximum concentrations allowed. Additives must be thoroughly assessed for safety before they can be permitted. Each permitted additive is assigned an E number signifying that it has been approved as safe. Consumer intakes of additives are calculated to make sure that they are within internationally agreed safe limits.

This seems fine, except that some adults and many children are extremely sensitive to all different kinds of additives and children especially like to eat the same kind of food very often. Therefore, chemicals will accumulate somewhere in the body. Apart from this, we know hardly anything about interaction of the innumerable chemicals in our food. Unfortunately, although governments do their best, the problem of food safety is now out of hand and many additives seem to do more harm than good.

Even if your child does not seem to be very sensitive to such substances and appears quite healthy, you never know what will happen in the long run. The accumulation of toxins may continue for some months, years or even longer before the body or the mind reacts, but most certainly some day there will be a reaction. Lung cancer breaks out after a person has been smoking for several decades, but there are other terrible and chronic diseases that need much less time to develop. We still know so little, but we know that we cannot play with fire too long before disaster strikes.

We seem to have forgotten which foods are really suitable for us. Children eat sweets and drink soft drinks and parents wonder why their little darlings are so restless and look so pale. We are used to this kind of food, but the human organism will never get used to it.

Now, let us take an open-minded and critical look at the entire picture of additives. Much that has been written on the subject is a conglomerate of truth and untruth, of logical and illogical criticism, or fanaticism. For example, not all additives are dangerous and sometimes industry has to use them. In the tropics it is not difficult to identify situations where staple food becomes potentially dangerous owing to spoilage through microbial action. Food spoils very fast in the tropics and as the population growth in these countries is enormous, some chemical preservatives are really needed. In that case it is important to make a choice of the best and least harmful preservatives.

However, the use of preservatives and other chemicals should always be kept within a certain framework and not used exclusively for financial gain. In our industrial countries, food does not spoil as fast as in the tropics. A few harmless preservatives should be permitted, but they should only exceptionally be added to foods or drinks consumed by children. Grown-ups usually have much more resistance to toxins than children and teenagers.

It is interesting to observe that most preservatives, colourings and other chemicals are not added to common daily food, but mainly to 'non-food' – to junk food or to sweets and soft drinks that harm us and our children. Such 'non-foods' and beverages do not contain any valuable nutrients and on top of that, unscrupulous and indifferent manufacturers add colourings and taste-enhancing chemicals so that they taste and look good. The witch in 'Snow White' did the same thing with the apple, but we seem to have learned nothing from this fairytale.

Americans allow over 10,000 additives into their food supply. The situation in Europe is not yet as bad, but as the pharmaceutical companies manufacturing additives are usually multinationals, European countries will soon follow. The average American eats 14 pounds of chemical additives per year. In addition to artificial chemical colourings, preservatives, flavourings, emulsifiers and anti-microbials, Americans consume on average 120 pounds of sugar and 8 pounds of salt per year. In Europe these figures are not much less.

Besides arthritis, clogged blood vessels and other 'civilisation diseases' (as I call the diseases that are prevalent in modern Western society), modern eating habits and countless food additives can cause behavioural problems in sensitive children. About one-quarter of all children in industrial countries suffer from attention deficit, hyperactivity, sleep disorders, emotional stress, nervousness, autism, obesity, tooth decay or diabetes, and the number increases every year.

The first junk food came originally from the United States and the first sweets and pastries probably came from Europe. Customs that are fashionable in the West always have their copycats in Eastern countries. For many years, people in those countries thought that everything coming from the West was best. Teenagers in faraway countries love to wear denim jeans. Technical progress was very helpful for many Eastern countries and at the beginning of the Westernising wave there was also great admiration for the medicine of the West. More and more patients were treated with antibiotics and other strong medication, while traditional medicine that had been used for thousands of years was relegated to the corner shop. However, now people have started realising that strong medicine is not only expensive, it is often very dangerous indeed. Things are changing, and many old remedies and treatments have come back into favour and are taught side by side with Western medicine.

It would not be too harmful if this was the only Western influence, but the Westernising tendency can also be seen in bad living, eating and drinking habits. For some decades hamburgers and hot-dogs have been eaten by millions of teenagers in those countries and millions of gallons of soft drinks are sold. At the same time, the children in these countries, who had always had a very strict education, have have changed their behaviour. The elder generation is shocked by the bad behaviour of the younger generation and in those countries the crime wave is increasing each month.

❧ *Chapter 18* ❧

INDIRECT FOOD ADDITIVES

Besides the additives mentioned in the last chapter, there are about 5,000 substances which are known as 'indirect additives'. These are, for example, substances that may come into contact with food as part of packaging or from processing equipment or substances that are used in some stage of the processing but afterwards are not needed any more. One can compare this to a wedding, whereby an official representative of the municipality is needed for the union, but afterwards his or her help is no longer needed.

In the USA the FDA has a long list of such substances. Some of these are natural and usually they are harmless. Others are not so harmless and many of them are man-made chemical substances. There are metals and metalloids, many different acids, as well as cobalt, copper, petroleum, asbestos, asphalt, borax and so on. Quite a few of these may be harmful or even poisonous to the human organism, but as long as this has not been proved absolutely, food containing them can still be sold.

Most people believe that the quantities used for 'refining' our food are so small that they can do no harm. Those responsible for our health do not seem to know that many such substances could have a toxic or even a lethal effect, even when diluted 100 or 1,000 times. Of course, the defence mechanisms of our body are able to render many of these toxins harmless. However, the defence mechanisms of any person who consumes the same foods or soft drinks over a long period will have to eliminate a growing amount of the same kind of harmful substances.

After some time elimination will stagnate and the toxins will accumulate in the body, in the nervous system and in the brain of the person in question. Children are generally far more sensitive to toxins than grown-ups and the brain is the most sensitive part of the body. Children do not read labels and so it is easy to deceive them when the industry uses taste and colouring chemicals to match their tastes.

❧ Chapter 19 ❧

DANGEROUS METALS

There is no escape possible any more. Our modern world is full of heavy metals: they are in the soil, in the air we breathe, in the water we drink and in most things that have to do with modern life. Heavy metals enter our body through our skin, through our lungs and through our digestive tract.

Heavy metals are very toxic and bioaccumulative: this means that they can accumulate in the human body. When too many toxins enter our body, our liver and other detoxifying organs are overburdened. Toxic metals are deposited in the walls of our blood vessels, in the lymphatic system, in our organs, in our connective tissues and in all the cells in our body, mainly our fat cells. After accumulating sometimes for many years or even decades, the health of the entire organism will be compromised. While some metal poisoning is still reversible in adults, in children it can interfere with normal development or cause brain damage.

Small children love to take almost everything in their mouths. They chew on their toys, on a little piece of cloth, on the windowsill in the subway, and even on painted walls and furniture. In that way lead and other toxic and dangerous metals enter directly into the organism of the child and this can be very dangerous considering the metallic avalanche of the past decades.

Morton Walker said that 'each person living in Western industrialised countries today is known to be at least 1,000 times more polluted with toxic metals and/or heavy metals than anyone who lived when Christ walked the earth'.

Where do all these toxic and heavy metals come from? From the earliest beginnings they were part of nature, but they did not threaten the health of the people, for hardly any metals were used at that time. When the Romans became rulers of the Western world of their time, Roman citizens started to use metals and other materials or substances they found in nature, in order to improve their living conditions. Just as the Egyptians and even older civilisations had done before, they made jewellery from precious stones and ordinary metals. But that was not all; Romans used copper, tin and lead for household and other appliances and most of their water pipes were made from lead. Their wine goblets and crockery were also made from heavy metals and they used powdered copper in order to improve the taste of their wine.

With the exception of some emperors, kings and noblemen in Egypt and in the Eastern countries, there were few people who used so many different metals as the Romans. It did them no good – some historians even believe that the fall of the Roman Empire had something to do with a slow self-poisoning of its inhabitants, due to the high toxicity of some of the metals they used. Maybe they are right.

What is happening in our time is still worse. Many different heavy and toxic metals have become part of our modern life. Many branches of industry use metals and mainly through the growth of industry they have been dispersed to every aspect of our life. A poor diet, lacking in many important nutrients, goes hand in hand with the use of heavy metals changing the biochemistry in which the brain functions. From the early morning until we go to sleep we are surrounded by many different toxic metals.

The number of babies born with a heavy load of toxins is escalating, and nobody seems to realise how much this has to do with toxic metals and with our lack of knowledge in this area. Small and sensitive children in particular are the victims of this ignorance. Children who have had an early exposure to lead and other heavy metals are likely to exhibit AD/HD symptoms like hyperactivity.

By and large, lead, mercury, aluminium, copper and cadmium are the most dangerous, and all day long we are in contact with these metals without realising the danger.

Lead is still being used in many industrial plants. We absorb lead by drinking contaminated water, or by breathing polluted air. Many old houses still have lead pipes. There may be lead in your toothpaste tube and that lead will be assimilated by the toothpaste and get into your organism. Newspaper ink contains lead, and it is also to be found in insecticides, in fungicides, in some commercial baby milk, in many different kinds of fish, in offal, in cosmetics, in hair colourings, in paper clips, in cooking utensils, in glassware, in lead paint, in wine, in cigarette smoke and in parks where children play. When you smoke a cigarette, you can relax while getting some nice lead arsenate, used in tobacco as an insecticide, into your lungs. Although the use of lead in cars is no longer permitted, exhaust fumes from cars can still endanger our health in other ways.

Some of the symptoms of lead poisoning are impotence, sterility, birth defects, insomnia, anaemia, muscle weakness, constipation or diarrhoea, headaches, depression, fatigue, irritability and so on. When only small quantities of lead accumulate in the body, a child may suffer from fatigue, growth problems, restlessness, muscle weakness, mental retardation, learning difficulties, loss of appetite, anorexia, confusion, impaired motor skill development, behaviour disorders, irritability and behaviour changes.

Mercury (thimerosal) can leak out from amalgam fillings. Mercury fillings become highly potent neurotoxins, easily absorbed by nerve cells. These toxins infiltrate the brain, as well as other parts of the body, within 24 hours. We may also find mercury in laxatives, cosmetics and prescription drugs. There is often mercury in fabric softeners. Mercury is even in some hepatitis B and DPT vaccines! Many large kinds of fish, like tuna or salmon, fresh or tinned, may contain mercury. Chemical fertilisers, pesticides, fungicides, water-based paints and even fluorescent light bulbs often contain mercury.

As a consequence of the accumulation of this metal, there is emotional instability, depression, fatigue, poor concentration, memory loss and hypertension. Mercury can cause kidney damage, tremors, loss of hearing and vision, sore gums, gingivitis and headaches. Even small quantities can provoke mental retardation, skin eruptions, chronic fatigue, learning disabilities, apathy, drowsiness, nervousness, chromosome damage and AD/HD in children. There is an interesting similarity between the symptoms of mercury poisoning and autism.

Removing amalgam fillings from your teeth can be dangerous if your dentist does not know how to go about it properly. A dentist who is really health-conscious will be sure to do so very carefully, so that as little mercury as possible enters into the bloodstream, from where it could get into the rest of the body.

Aluminium can be found in many deodorants, in cooking ware and in construction materials. Kettles can be made from aluminium, copper or other metals, and the table salt we use for our egg in the morning contains some aluminium in order to keep the salt dry. We still use aluminium in aerosol sprays and kitchen foil. Aluminium is even used in our food, in the emulsifier for cheese processing, in baking powder, in salt, to prevent humidity, in beer and soft-drink cans, and in pharmaceutical drugs, such as anti-acids and many others. The aluminium silicates from aerosol sprays can be directly transported through nerve connections from the nose into the brain and deposited in the most sensitive areas. According to a report in the *Lancet* (1989), many infant formulas contain aluminium. Human breast milk may contain 5–20 micrograms of aluminium per litre, but some formulas based on cows' milk contain 20 times as much, and soy-based formulas contain 100 times as much. Breast milk is still the safest milk by far.

Aluminium can cause headaches, brain degeneration, senile dementia and gastritis. In small children it may be the cause of gas, colic, motor and behavioural dysfunction, skin rashes and nervousness. The aluminium content of the brain of patients with dementia, in particular Alzheimer's disease, is greatly elevated compared to normal levels.

Aluminium is known to inhibit and reduce an important co-factor in the synthesis of many neurotransmitters. It also promotes acute psychotic conditions by making the blood-brain barrier more permeable to ingested neurotoxins.

Copper levels in the blood rise when zinc levels drop, as happens in females the week before their period and when on contraceptive pills. Copper levels also rise in both sexes when sugar is eaten. Copper comes from birth-control pills, copper water pipes, water heaters, pesticides, from brewery equipment, from salt, alcoholic beverages, from meats (here it is used as a growth enhancer) and from soya beans, in which levels are very high.

While copper is an essential trace mineral needed by our body, exposure to too great a quantity of copper may over-stimulate the brain and cause insufficiency of zinc, hair loss, anaemia, arthritis, insomnia, poor concentration, irritability, hypertension, postpartum psychosis, toxaemia in pregnancy, inflammation of the liver, cystic fibrosis (high copper levels) and in children digestive disorders, colic and behavioural problems. In schizophrenics copper levels are usually very high.

When the excess of copper has been removed by chelation there is usually a rapid improvement. While eliminating copper from the body, as a reaction to the cleansing efforts you may get acne. Acne will break out where the copper stores are being depleted, for example around your mouth, your neck or your chest. When these surplus metals are gone from the body, the acne disappears. Zinc helps to counteract some of the harmful effects of copper.

Cadmium is still found in some water pipes, and in cigarettes, fertilisers, soft-drink dispensers, old dental fillings, refined foods and plated containers, and it can leak from plastics. It can cause emphysema, kidney and liver damage, nephritis, abdominal cramps, colic, slow healing (because of a zinc deficiency), anaemia, acne and hypertension, and is known as a zinc antagonist. The cadmium in cigarette smoke is very dangerous. It is not only toxic for the smoker, but also for the non-smoker, especially children.

When children suffer from problems such as ADD, AD/HD, hyperactivity, autism, learning disabilities, irritability and other mental problems, as well as allergies, tummy-aches and constipation, the cause is an accumulation of heavy and toxic metals in combination with other negative factors and influences.

Vanadium is relatively high in milk, egg white, gelatine and shell-fish. It is a heavy metal, which in trace amounts seems to be essential for us. When vanadium is elevated in the blood and the hair, severe depression may occur. In that case a supplement of ascorbic acid can be very helpful. Vanadium can prevent the transport of sodium across cell membranes. This means that the sodium content inside the cells becomes too high and cells cannot build up the full electric potential for proper functioning. If blood pressure is low, this can produce apathy, memory impairment and social withdrawal.

❧ Chapter 20 ❧

SALICYLATES

Salicylates are chemicals that occur naturally in many plants. They act as preservatives to delay rotting and protect against harmful bacteria, fungi and insects. They are stored in the bark, leaves, roots and seeds of plants. Salicylates can be found naturally in many different foods and their compounds are used in medical drugs and in many different products.

Acetylsalicylic acid is the chemical name for aspirin. The naturally occurring precursor for aspirin is salicylic acid, which is found in the bark of willow trees. Salicylic acid causes gastric distress, so its chemical relative is used more often. Chemically it is synthesised from the aromatic benzene ring, which can either occur naturally or be made artificially.

In medicine salicylates are used to relieve pain and reduce fever. Aspirin is the most commonly used remedy containing salicylates, but there are at least 100 similar remedies. These often help to relieve symptoms caused by arthritis and other rheumatic diseases. Sometimes physicians prescribe them in cases of heart problems. However, salicylates do not cure, and will help you only as long as you continue to take them.

Drugs that contain salicylates include analgesics (painkillers), muscle relaxants, cough mixtures, antacids, cold and flu medication and acne lotions.

Salicylates, or acetylsalicylic acid, can be found all over, in artificial flavours and natural flavours used in foods, spice flavourings and products, beverages, sweets, chewing gum, breath mints, some prescription medications, toothpaste, mouthwash, cough drops, perfumes, deodorants and dishwashing liquids. Disinfectants and air fresheners also contain salicylic acid derivatives.

There are many over-the-counter remedies that contain salicylates. Salicylates also can be found in artificial food colourings and flavourings, such as peppermint and strawberry.

Salicylic acid is permitted as a preservative in adhesives, used for food packaging, in cardboard containers that will be in contact with foods and for sealing food containers. Therefore salicylic acid may occur as a 'migration compound' that gets into food from packaging materials.

Salicylates are known to block the information of substances known as protaglandins (PGs). Hyperactive children might be deficient in PGs, notably PGE1, which is formed from a specific fatty acid, dihomo-gama-linolenic acid (DGLA). These fatty acids cannot be made by the body, but must be taken in via foods. The most important polyunsaturated acid is linolic acid. This is a major constituent of vegetable oils like sunflower and safflower oil (buy these only as cold-pressed oils). Evening Primrose oil is extremely useful.

However, some children do not seem to be able to convert essential fatty acids to PGE1, which is crucial in the control of the immune system and behaviour. They cannot convert them because of a lack of zinc, vitamin B3 and B6, and vitamin C.

Salicylate sensitivity is the body's inability to handle more than a certain amount of salicylates at any one time. Some adults and children have a low level of tolerance to salicylates and may get symptoms that are dose-related. The tolerated amount varies from one person to another. This is a good example of food intolerance. For people with a family history of food intolerance, salicylates are more likely to cause problems than any other food chemical.

Salicylates in food are usually not concentrated enough to do us any harm. The liver processes the tiny amounts to salicylate tagged with glycine, which apparently makes such substances less offensive. However, when salicylates from lipstick or make up are applied to skin, lips or mouth membranes, they are rapidly absorbed and go directly to the kidneys, without the benefit of first passing through the liver, where they would be detoxified. When herbal medicines or plant concentrates are taken by mouth, there are often sufficient salicylates to overwhelm the liver's capacity to glycinate and when this happens the kidneys can be harmed.

Salicylate sensitivity can manifest itself in many ways. For example, asthma, breathing difficulties, congestion, fatigue, headaches, hyperactivity, itchy skin, rashes or hives, itchy, watery, or swollen eyes, lack of concentration or memory, mouth ulcers, persistent cough, sinusitis, stomach-aches or upsets, an urgent need to pass water, or bed-wetting. Salicylates can also cause chronic urticaria, eczema, asthma, nasal polyps, sinusitis and rhino conjunctivitis.

Symptoms of overdose in children are behavioural changes, drowsiness or tiredness (severe), fast or deep breathing, trouble in sleeping, nervousness or jitters (this only applies to products also containing caffeine, like cola drinks).

SALICYLATES IN FOODS

Raw food, dried food and juices contain higher levels of salicylates than cooked food. The salicylate content in foods is highest in unripe fruit and decreases as the fruit ripens. All fruit and vegetables should be ripe and thickly peeled before eating. Salicylates are often concentrated just under the skin of fruit and vegetables, and in the outer leaves of vegetables.

If you are sensitive to salicylates, try to avoid foods such as the following, which have a high salicylate content: plums (tinned), raspberries (fresh), cherries, peppers, almonds, peppermint tea, prunes (tinned), strawberries (fresh), grapes (juice and sultanas), broccoli, citrus fruits, tomatoes, peanuts, honey and mint-flavoured toothpaste. All fresh meat, fish, shellfish, poultry, eggs, dairy products, cereals and bread are low in salicylates.

With society's increasing consumption of processed foods, most people will ingest the majority of their foodborne salicylates from synthetic additives, especially flavourings. Because at least some salicylates readily pass through the skin, any present in suntan lotion, cosmetics, perfumes or topical creams could further boost exposure.

In a recent study, salicylates appeared in the top six problem chemicals for each major symptom:

- Behavioural problems (salicylates, preservatives, nitrates, amines, MSG, colours)
- Eczema (salicylates, preservatives, nitrates, colours, amines, MSG)
- Irritable bowel (MSG, salicylates, nitrates, preservatives, amines, colours)
- Lethargy/impairment of memory and concentration (salicylates, nitrates, preservatives, MSG, amines, colours)
- Migraine (nitrates, preservatives, salicylates, MSG, amines, colours)

The most effective way of treating this intolerance appears to be the Feingold Diet, which removes salicylates from the diet. This seems to be highly effective in decreasing the symptoms of AD/HD in many children. As many as 25 per cent of all children appear to be sensitive to salicycates.

Discovering if your child is sensitive to salicylates, is allergic to different foods or has food incompatibilities is a very difficult task, and it is almost impossible to cut out all sources. The best you can do is write down, every day, everything your child eats and drinks. You should also take note of the time he or she ate, and write down every symptom and the time at which this symptom began. Probably you will find a pattern, and there will be a correlation of eating and drinking certain foods or drinks and symptoms. You will soon know what foods you have to cut out.

Later it might be possible to reintroduce some of the foods your child likes, but you will have to go very slowly, starting with the smallest quantities of only one food at a time. Often most foods can be tolerated again after some weeks or months, but sometimes it takes a few years. However, they should only be eaten in small amounts and provided that not too many of the foods that formerly were a problem for your child are eaten at any one time.

Chapter 21

A LACK OF NUTRIENTS

Many children suffering from hyperactivity, restlessness, aggressiveness, depression, autism and different behavioural problems have a lack of several important nutrients. Sometimes these children may also have a toxic surplus of some other natural or unnatural substances.

Although this is not always the case and there are many variations to be seen, these children are often low in calcium, magnesium, boron, vitamin B6, vitamin B12 and zinc. They are often high in folic acid, sodium, selenium, potassium, copper and iron.

A lack of certain nutrients is, however, not always due to the fact that food containing such nutrients is missing in the diet of the child. Sometimes these nutrients, because of a lack of the necessary enzymes or for other reasons, cannot be assimilated by the body. As yet we know very little of all the complicated processes in our body.

If you cannot find out what is causing the problem, the best way to help your child is to go to a physician or naturopath who knows about orthomolecular therapy (see Chapter 29); they will probably recommend that a hair test be done. This is the best way to find out what nutrients your child lacks, or what surplus toxins are interfering with normal processes in their body and mind.

Often when I tell parents that it is not advisable to give their baby, toddler or child cows' milk, they ask me where their children should get calcium from instead. I tell them that they can get plenty of calcium from vegetables, nuts, sesame seeds, dried fruit, figs, dates and that plums especially have lots of calcium. The type of calcium from this kind of food is far superior in quality and much easier to assimilate and digest than the calcium from cows' milk.

A lack of folic acid and B12 is often mentioned in reporting psychiatric illness and behavioural problems. There have been hundreds of articles written about this and much clinical research done on different groups of children with behavioural problems. The magnesium, zinc, copper, iron and calcium levels of the blood plasma of the child should be examined and urine and hair tests done. The average concentration of all trace elements is usually lower compared with trace elements in healthy children. Most children eat too few natural carbohydrates; often this can cause depression.

Children often have a lack of fatty acids and after a while there should be a great improvement when the children take evening primrose oil or omega-3 fatty acids regularly. These omega-3 fatty acids are known to be safe, natural mood stabilisers. They can be found in salmon, mackerel, tuna, sardines and other deep-sea, cold-water fish. Fish oils have no side-effects besides occasional light indigestion.

In the case of behavioural problems one should focus on a well-balanced diet, including plenty of leafy greens for folic acid, and bananas, avocado, chicken and wholegrains for vitamin B6. All children should drink plenty of water, at least six glasses a day. Good, fresh water should be kept in glass containers or bottles, never in plastic containers or bottles. Herbal teas should be prepared with this water and cooking water should also be high quality.

❧ Chapter 22 ❧

NOISE

Compared to 50 years ago, noise levels have increased tremendously. The world in which our children live is becoming noisier and noisier. In many households, televisions and audio equipment are turned on for the entire day, the phone rings, people are shouting and there are traffic noises from outside, creating a constantly noisy environment.

Because children do not possess such good coping responses as adults and are less able to control their environment, they are more affected by noise than adults. Noise pollution can pose a potential risk to young children.

Noise level standards set by the Occupational Safety and the Health Administration (ASHA) are expressed in decibels, 'dB', indicating the noise level a human being can normally cope with. The noise level for the average citizen seems to be around 75dB, but we should never forget that in small children the sense of hearing is far more delicate.

When we as adults are continually exposed to a slightly higher noise level, for example of 85dB, it will eventually harm our hearing. If the noise level is still higher, for example 15 minutes' exposure at 115dB, this is considered dangerous to hearing.

Some toys designed to stimulate children are dangerously loud. For the infant or child whose arms are shorter than those of an adult, and who listens to such toys close to their small ear, the risk is even greater. Potential sources of hearing impairment and psychological problems in children are: toddlers' noisy toys, firecrackers, power tools, musical instruments, walk- and discmans. Certain rattles and squeaky toys are measured at sound levels as high as 110dB. Musical toys, such as electric guitars, drums and horns, emit sounds as high as 120dB. Toy phones for small children are measured at between 123 and 129dB. Toys which are designed to amplify the voice are measured at up to 135dB.

In 1982 the United States National Research Council issued a warning that pregnant mothers should avoid working in noisy environments. The hearing of an embryo is already developed after about four weeks and the foetus can hear different tones, especially high-pitched voices. The foetal ear is a very sensitive instrument that can easily be harmed by loud noises. Premature babies have such a sensitive sense of hearing that loud noises can harm them physically as well as mentally. Physically there is the potential risk of weakened blood-vessel walls of the brain, growth retardation and serious hearing impairment. There may also be sleeping problems, and the emotional development of the child may be slowed down.

Physical and psychological problems always come together. One typical example for this is the link between mental stress and stomach ulcers.

For preschool and school-age children noise and intrusive sounds can have the following effects: a change in the heart rhythm; a rise in blood pressure; excessive hormonal excretions; stress; hearing impairment; cramps; inner tension; sleeping and emotional problems.

Children all react in different ways to stress like loud noises. Most children have a tendency to start screaming and yelling themselves in order to drown out other noises. Although we do not realise it, noisy children are often extremely sensitive to noise. However, there are other children who prefer to hide in a corner or retreat within themselves when confronted with too much noise. Noisy children will soon show signs of hyperactivity and restlessness if they cannot cope with the level of noise around them, but children who are generally more quiet will become extremely so. If noises accelerate and the stress becomes intolerable, the entire personality of these children seems to undergo a change.

Never before has this world been so unsuitable for children.

They all deserve a happy childhood, but as a consequence of the combination of a toxic environment, the destruction of natural habitats, toxic and worthless food, sugary unhealthy drinks, drugs, alcohol, stressed and frightened adults and far too much noise everywhere, only a few children are still more or less healthy. It is still unknown to what extent hyperactivity, aggressive behaviour, helplessness and autism are consequences of noise exposure. However, it is certain, that in combination with other negative factors, excessive noise plays an important role. Current knowledge strongly suggests that over-stimulation through too much noise hinders normal emotional development in children of all ages.

Noise in the classroom and outside has been associated with lower attentiveness and responsibility, problems with speech perception and reading acquisition. The level of noise confusion at home, as well as traffic noises from outside, can have a great impact on early childhood development.

Noise can affect the temperament and social interactions of children, and increases the susceptibility of the child to the harmful effects of other environmental influences. The evidence on links between noise pollution and children's health is strong enough to warrant monitoring programmes at schools and pre-schools to protect children from the effects of noise. Children may feel helpless in the face of pervasive, consistent noise over which they have no control.

Studies on the adverse effects of environmental noise on mental health cover a variety of symptoms, including anxiety, emotional stress, headaches, instability, argumentativeness, changes in mood and an increase in social conflicts, as well as general psychiatric disorders such as neurosis, psychosis and hysteria.

When children become teenagers, they are so used to loud noise that they feel lost in quiet surroundings. Loud noises can be intoxicating and can act like a drug. Teenagers or adults who use a walkman listen on average for 24 hours or more per week to very loud music of about 100dB, which enters the ear directly.

Several studies have demonstrated a relationship between noise and aggressive acts. The sound of motorbikes and mopeds gives their owners a feeling of power and strength, while at the same time they may become aggressive and lose their sense of judgement and caution. Taking alcohol or drugs at the same time can have disastrous consequences. As the traffic in large urban areas and many other places is constantly increasing, noise pollution has become a very serious problem.

Children need quiet time at home, to create, learn and relax. If we want our children to live in a peaceful world, we must first offer them opportunities for quiet relaxation, to meditate and to dream. All our senses should be coordinated and function in harmony. Dr Alfred Tomatis believes that the problems I mention in this book are partly a consequence of a disharmony of the senses. We do not hear only with our ears; we also react to sounds that are transmitted to the inner ear by way of vibrations through the bones. Dr Tomatis and other scientists are convinced that children and adults suffering from ADD, autism and other behaviour deviations do not know how to pick up sounds directly through the external part of the ear, where these sounds are filtered before entering the inner ear. For these patients the continuous attacks of sound waves directly to the inner ear mean a constant stress situation. This harms the sensitive nervous system, especially in young children. In the Tomatis Centres in Europe and the USA children and grown-ups are taught how to use their sense of hearing in the right way. Many former patients are very enthusiastic about this music and sound therapy. Preferably this method should be combined with other natural healing methods.

Many children do not know what a wonderful experience it is to be outside in the country and listen to all the sounds of nature. The League for the Hard of Hearing introduces school-age children, parents and teachers to the delights of everyday sounds and recommends a wonderful book, *Listen to the Raindrops* by Arline Bronzaft.

❧ Chapter 23 ❧

E NUMBERS AND OTHER DANGERS

The following information is intended only to give some basic guidelines on E numbers and other additives. My recommendations are based on information from health organisations in many countries. I do not claim that the information in this chapter is all-encompassing, or even particularly extensive. My objective is simply to open your eyes to the fact that our modern food is filled with so many toxic substances that it can seriously endanger our health and above all the health of our children.

Many 'natural food colours' can be produced synthetically and are not always safe in large doses. They are, for example: E 101, 101a, 100, 120, 140, 141, 160a, 160b, 160c, 160d, 160f, 161b, 162 and 163. They can be found for example in curcumin, chlorophyl, beetroot juice, carotine and tomato pigment.

Here is a list of the additives (E numbers) you should try to avoid.

FOOD ADDITIVES
E 102, 104, 107, 110, 120, 122, 129 (123 was banned in America in 1976), 132, 133, 133, 142, 150, 151, 153, 154, 155 (some of these are still used in the United States).

Food colourings can cause wakefulness in children, can affect asthmatics, cause shortness of breath, itching, nettle rash, a runny nose, blurred vision, gastric upsets and produce reactions in aspirin-sensitive people. It is possible that they affect the thyroid gland, and they have been implicated in minimal brain dysfunction in children.

These additives can be found in confectionery, fruit juices, cordials, soft drinks, tinned fruit and vegetables, fruit-flavoured yoghurt, sauces, pickles, hot chocolate mix, packet soup, jelly crystals, pre-packaged sandwich fillings, marzipan, fruit-flavoured fillings, glacé cherries, Scotch eggs and custard mix, and many other foods.

E 132 is a preservative that may cause vomiting, nausea or high blood pressure and should be avoided by people who have a history of allergy. It is present in biscuits and confectionery.

E 151, 154 and 155 are used in the UK but banned in several other countries.

E 160b has some adverse reactions, like nettle rash and specific edema in heart patients.

E 200–03: sorbates (containing sorbic acid) are a possible skin irritant, so sensitive people should avoid them. They can be found in many food products: mixed dried fruit, sausagemeat, beer, cider, fruit juice, some jams, gelatine, wine, vinegar, brewed soft drinks and non-tinned tomato juice.

E 210 is a preservative that should be avoided by asthmatics and may be responsible for some neurological disorders. It can be found in cordials, chilli paste, soft drinks, fruit juice, dips and non-tinned tomato juice.

E 211 and 212 should be avoided by asthmatics and can be found in the same foods listed for E 210 (211 is not used in the United States).

E 213, 218, 220, 221, 222 and 223 are preservatives that may cause adverse reactions in asthmatics and aspirin-sensitive people. It can cause gastric irritations, diarrhoea and allergic skin reactions, and can be found in fruit juice, cordials, cider, dried fruit, dehydrated peas, syrups, flavoured toppings, uncooked prawns and shrimps.

E 220–28 are sulphites that may trigger asthma attacks and allergic reactions, and could destroy vitamin B1. Sulphites can be found in pickles and in products mentioned for E 213.

E 230, 231, 232, 233 can cause skin problems.

E 223 and 252 have been known to cause allergic reactions and can be found in bread and flour products.

E 249–52 are nitrates and nitrites. (E 250 and 251 are not used in the US.) They are not permitted in foods for children. Nitrites can affect the blood's ability to transport oxygen. They can be dangerous. Possible sources are: tinned, cured and pickled meat, manufactured, processed meat, pressed meat, uncooked, fermented, manufactured meat sausages, raw ham, Italian-type ham, smoked meat products. Naturally high levels of nitrites can be found in beetroot, celery and spinach.

E 280–83 are preservatives. They may cause migraine and are found in bread and flour products.

E 310–21 are antioxidants (also indicated as preservatives). Many of them should not be permitted in foods intended for infants. They cause adverse reactions in aspirin-sensitive people and asthmatics. They can be found in edible fats, spreads, lard, drippings and margarine, in pecan and walnut kernels, and in all kinds of food as a result of absorption from food wrappings.

E 355: adipic acid (often included in flavourings). This may cause seizures in those unable to metabolise it.

E 338, 339, 340, 341, 450, 461, 463, 465, and 466 may provoke digestive problems.

E420 and 421. Large amounts can cause diarrhoea.

E 469 (sodium caseinate) should be avoided when sensitive to milk. It is found in cheese. E 620–35 are flavour enhancers often used in Chinese food. Their ingredient is monosodium glutamate [MSG]. This should not be permitted in foods manufactured for children and infants. It is found in sauces, packet soups, flavoured noodles and different condiments. MSG acts as a vasodilator and may trigger migraines. It is not permitted in Australia.

The above-mentioned side-effects from food additives are only part of the picture. The list is far from complete – many side-effects are unknown and perhaps always will be, as we cannot predict what after-effects the accumulation and interactions of all these chemicals that disturb the natural balance and functioning of our metabolism will have in the future. What we are doing to our food and to the health of millions of people is irresponsible, but there are financial and other interests that seem to be stronger than the wish to do the right thing.

We can only try to live as healthily as possible ourselves, and that means in the first place avoiding all known health-endangering products, such as for example:

> Pre-made soups, sauces, boullions or custards
> Pastries with fruit or fruit flavouring
> Yoghurt with fruit or fruit flavouring
> Fruit/vegetable juices
> All processed luncheon meats
> Crisps
> Fast food
> Soft drinks
> Most restaurant food
> Vitamin A (palmitate). This may include E 321, 320 and 319
> Refined oil (for the same reasons as vitamin A)

Much flavouring may be artificial, made of hundreds of chemical compounds. 'Natural' flavouring may contain salicylates or MSG. Please note that vanillin is an artificial flavouring. It may also be called 'vanilla flavouring'. Look for 'pure vanilla' in the ingredients instead.

Do you know that about one-third of the crude oil in the western world goes into the manufacturing of our clothing, cosmetics, shampoos, detergents, perfumes, paints, plastics, pesticides and – most important – our food? Whatever we do, we come into contact with the by-products of crude oil and some of us, especially children, have difficulty coping with these powerful substances.

Do not purchase foods containing the following ingredients for your children:

> MSG
> Gelatine
> Calcium caseinate
> Hydrolysed vegetable protein
> Textured protein
> Monopotassium glutamate

Hydrolysed plant protein
Yeast extract
L-cystine
Glutamate
Autolysed plant protein
Yeast food or nutrient
Glutamic acid
Sodium caseinate
Autolysed yeast
Natural flavours
Spices/seasonings

All this may seem terribly complicated, but it is important to realise that most problems stem from completely altered foods. Natural foods that are not treated in any way and do not contain additives will hardly ever do harm.

We have to learn again how to eat natural food and enjoy it. Diets like the Feingold Diet will teach us how to help our children. As Surgeon General Burney said about 30 years ago:

> Must we wait until we prove every link in the causation?
> In protecting health absolute proof comes late. To wait for
> it is to invite disaster or to prolong suffering unnecessarily.
> I submit that those things within man's power to control
> which impact upon the individual in a negative way, which
> infringe upon his sense of integrity, and interrupt his
> pursuit of fulfilment, are hazards to public health.

It is sad to note that today not only people but also governments have continued to lack the will to remedy most of these problems and have totally denied that many additives are perilous to people's health and well-being.

DIETARY RECOMMENDATIONS
Eat a wholefood diet high in protein and complex carbohydrates. Cut down on sugar and simple carbohydrates. Cut back on processed junk foods high in additives and food colourings.

The Hyperactive Children's Support Group of Great Britain recommends that the following food additives be avoided:

Tartrazine
Sunset Yellow
Benzoic acid
Amaranth
Red 2G
Brilliant FCF
Carmine
Quinoline Yellow
FCFV
Carmoic acid
Sulphur dioxide
Potassium nitrate
BHT
Caramel
Cochineal
Sodium benzoate
Sodium nitrate
BHA
Indigo

Governmental and many private organisations also have lists of different foods and E numbers that they recommend or disapprove of. There are extensive lists on the websites of many health organisations. Some of these lists may be exaggerated and others too lenient, but they all serve as a very serious warning that we should stop tinkering with our food. The consequences of what we have done wrong up to now are already showing, especially in our youth, and they are very frightening.

Chapter 24

MODERN MEDICINE

There is nothing intrinsically wrong with pharmacological medicine, but the way in which it is used is often wrong. Orthodox medicine is wonderful in an emergency and has saved thousands of lives, but a physician who prescribes antibiotics or other strong remedies for someone who has flu or another minor ailment makes a great mistake. This kind of medicine should be used exclusively for emergencies. If you have read the previous chapters, you will know that most chemical substances are toxic and can be very dangerous. You should also know why these substances were developed in the first place and why they are so toxic.

It all began with Pasteur, the great nineteenth-century French scientist. In 1865 Pasteur discovered the link between bacteria and disease. He was convinced that germs were the cause of all diseases. If the bacteria was killed, all diseases would be cured. Based on this idea, scientists developed strong chemical substances by which germs could be killed. Pharmaceutical companies shot up like mushrooms and thousands of men found a new scope of work.

Although dangerous infections were curtailed and these drugs did wonders in case of emergencies, illness did not disappear and many new and chronic diseases developed. Pasteur had not found the right solution and even he admitted at the end of his life that he had been wrong; that germs were only the consequence of the disease and not their cause. The environment of the germs was far more important, as germs could only live and multiply under certain conditions, which they found in already diseased surroundings inside a human body. If a person was healthy germs could not multiply. With the strong drugs that are being developed by pharmaceutical companies, germs can be killed and symptoms can be suppressed, but these drugs cannot heal.

Most scientists are of the opinion that the chemical substances and products we use in our laboratories and in our daily life are identical to the components we find in nature, for example in vegetables and fruit. However, a slight discrepancy invalidates this way of thinking. In nature it is almost impossible to find any of these chemical substances by themselves. Most of them are part of a symbiosis, a composition of many different substances, and every one of these substances has to fulfil its own special task. This can be compared to all the different instruments in an orchestra, which together make beautiful music.

Over the course of millions of years, through trial and error, by choosing and combining uncountable substances, nature created all life on earth. Everything natural that we eat and can digest is a composition of many known, and many still unknown, substances. By contrast, most of the chemicals we have used in all aspects of our life for the last 50 to100 years are single chemicals which in nature do not exist by themselves. When we use such chemicals for the fabrication of building materials, cars, bicycles, household articles, clothing and thousands of other things, it means progress and makes life easier for us. This seems okay, but in the last century we have become far too conceited with our scientific knowledge. Within a very short time-span, we have started trying to undo all the work nature has done for millions of years.

Like children who want to know how everything functions, we take any kind of natural composition apart in order to use the different pieces for our own goals. This may be right when it serves a technical or other material purpose, but where human health is concerned we have to be extremely careful.

The components of a natural chemical composition always belong together, like the instruments in an orchestra, but only a few people seem to realise this. A child who wants to know why a clock ticks tries to take the clock apart, to disassemble it as far as possible to find out what is ticking inside, thereby destroying the clock;

scientists do exactly the same thing. When the chief executives of a pharmaceutical company hear about plants growing somewhere on the planet that seem to have healing properties, they buy the plants and take them apart in order to find out what bit of the plant has healing properties. They do not seem to understand that the secret of those healing properties lies in the combination of many different substances in that plant. They are convinced that there is one special substance in the plant which has healing properties. If they are able to separate this special substance from the other components of the plant in question, the first step in manufacturing a new drug has been taken. After several years of testing, cleansing, sterilising and stabilising, as well as other manipulations, and of course after receiving the blessing of the health officials, their newest product is ready for sale.

For these remedies to sell and make money, the pharmaceutical company depends mainly on the power of their sales promotion. Formerly most decisions about such medication were left in the hands of physicians, working for the company in question. Nowadays almost all such decisions are made by their sales department.

It should be clear that such a drug could never be used to heal any disease. It can only suppress the symptoms. These drugs are so highly concentrated that they will paralyse the self-healing forces that are desperately needed during the recovery process in every kind of disease. As such drugs are extremely toxic, we can be sure that there will always be some more or less dangerous side-effects. Many of these side-effects will be treated with other drugs and the patient will be caught up in a vicious circle from which some people are never able to escape.

Tranquillisers and similar medications are sold in unbelievable quantities. Parents, teachers and other people who are responsible for a child may heave a sigh of relief when their behaviour improves, but many children taking such medication become like zombies and their normal mental reactions are totally suppressed. After a longer time all these remedies have more or less serious side-effects and anyone can very easily become dependent on such a drug; withdrawal often means hell.

If your physician prescribes medication for your mentally disturbed child, you should realise what it means and what risks you will be taking. The side-effects of these drugs can be so bad that the former symptoms were easier to bear and the parents become desperate. Before accepting that your child should take tranquillisers or other mind-altering medication, you should know that every year new and better ways to help such children are found. Do not make the wrong decision – you might regret it for the rest of your life.

❧ Chapter 25 ❧

RITALIN AND OTHER STRONG DRUGS

Each year more Ritalin and other powerful drugs are prescribed. The production of Ritalin, the most common prescription for AD/HD, increased 700 per cent between 1985 and 1998. Some five million children in industrial countries are taking anti-depressants, while anti-psychotic prescriptions have shot up by 268 per cent for youths.

These prescriptions run into many thousands for ADD or AD/HD, especially for hyperactive children. The list of side-effects is long and serious. We do not know the long-term effects of these and other drugs on children. Such drugs always create side-effects and these are often worse than the disease they are prescribed for. At worst, death can result from burst blood vessels in the brain or heart failure can occur. Many of these drugs are prescribed even for very young children and some kids even take twice the prescribed dose.

Dr Robert Mendelsohn, the author of *How to Raise a Healthy Child – in Spite of your Doctor*, says about Ritalin that apart from nervousness and insomnia and various and often serious skin diseases, there can be *necrotising vasculitis* (destruction of the blood vessels) and *thrombocytopenic purpura* (a serious blood-clotting disorder), anorexia, nausea, dizziness, palpitations, headache, dyskinesia (impairment of voluntary muscle movement), drowsiness, blood pressure and pulse changes, rapid heartbeat, angina (spasmodic attacks of intense heart pain), irregular heartbeat, abdominal pain, weight loss during prolonged therapy and so on. This information about the side-effects comes straight from the manufacturer of Ritalin and it is unbelievable that a great many physicians prescribe it and are still able to sleep at night.

Trusting and faithful supporters of strong medication believe that drugs such as Ritalin boost the capacity of the children to inhibit and regulate impulsive behaviour. What really happens is that such drugs paralyse the natural physical and mental processes in the bodies of these children, who cannot get rid of their aggression any more. Therefore it seems that their behaviour is improving, and that their mental and physical problems have abated. However, nothing could be farther from the truth. As soon as the children stop taking their medication, the symptoms come back right away and are usually worse than ever.

After taking these drugs for some time, children are unable to show any reactions and become very docile, reacting and often behaving like zombies. The claim that Ritalin improves the capacity for learning has never been proved.

Although the original hyperactivity or other behavioural problems of children taking strong medication cannot be detected any more, the original problem stays the same – there is never a cure. Believers in therapy with strong medication tell us that the day is not far off when genetic testing for AD/HD may become available and at last a cure will be found. New and even stronger medication, with still more dangerous side-effects, will be found. All those medicaments will be tested and tried on human guinea pigs. Poor children . . .

Pharmaceutical companies will have a greater turnover. However, the most important culprits, the toxins in our environment and in our food, will probably not be investigated more thoroughly or even mentioned. Already at one-hundredth of the lethal dose, the side-effects of these amphetamines can be detected, and that is a sign that such medication is far too strong.

CONVENTIONAL TREATMENT FOR HYPERACTIVITY

Ritalin (Methylphenidate), an amphetamine, is the most commonly prescribed medication for hyperactivity. This is what its manufacturers, Novartis Pharmaceuticals, say about their star medication:

> Ritalin calms the nerves and at the same time enhances the ability of a hyperactive child to pay attention. Ritalin can be taken when needed, so that a child need not take it, for example, on weekends or during vacations, when all that extra energy can find an outlet. Be sure, however, that you check with your doctor before taking your child off this medication. Potential side-effects of Ritalin include insomnia, decreased appetite, weight loss, slowed growth, increased heart rate and blood pressure, and an initial period of increased tearfulness and irritability.

Although Ritalin is the best-known suppressive amphetamine, there are a few other drugs that are regularly prescribed.

Peoline (Cylert) is a central nervous system stimulant that is often prescribed for hyperactivity. This medication enhances nerve impulse transmissions in the brain. It can cause insomnia.

Dexedrine (dextroamphetamine) is another medication sometimes prescribed for hyperactivity. This drug is a stimulant, but has the same paradoxical calming effect as Ritalin, as well as similar side-effects.

Triclic anti-depressant drugs, such as desipiramine or nortriptyline (pamelor), are less frequently prescribed. They are used mainly when an underlying depression is suspected.

Thiordazine (Mellaril) is a major tranquilliser that may be resorted to if a child is extremely aggressive, and then only in the most difficult situations.

The increased activity and short attention span of the child with AD/HD have led to the use of stimulant drugs such as Ritalin to control behaviour. Paradoxically, these medications work to 'slow down' the AD/HD child. Unfortunately, they are potentially harmful and act merely to mask symptoms without getting to the core of the problem.

Early intervention and successful treatment of AD/HD have become even more important in light of recent studies that predict these children face greater problems as adults. Evidence is mounting that children with AD/HD are at higher risk of depression, restlessness, alcoholism and anti-social behaviour as adults.

Chapter 26

CHILD PSYCHIATRY

In the United States, psychiatric counselling is very much in fashion. Many people have a 'shrink', and when they feel they cannot cope with their problems, they go there in the hope that it will help. It is quite rare for people now to take time to sort out their own troubles; many are of the opinion that somebody who has studied psychiatry for many years is better equipped to deal with them. It is a typical modern delusion that mental help is something that comes in jars at the health-food shop. Psychiatric help is very expensive; it may cost thousands, the treatment may take many years and most problems cannot be solved that way, because often the underlying causes are not recognised.

A friend of mine has a little son who was hyperactive from the age of two and had terrible tantrums. Everyone said that the child would probably grow out of it when he got older. However, a couple of years later his tantrums and hyperactivity had become much worse. His mother visited half a dozen of specialists who gave her advice and prescribed different kinds of tranquillisers, but the conduct of her son did not show any improvement. On the contrary, their recommendations seemed to do more harm than good.

Being dead tired, and at last responding to the urgent pleas of her husband and her own parents, my friend decided to take her son to see a child psychiatrist. Until then she had always said she did not want to take such a step, because she felt absolutely sure that her son was not crazy, but that there was something else bothering him. After she made this decision, she tried to find the right psychiatrist, something that turned out to be very difficult. Therefore she came to me for advice and I told her the following – there are many different schools of psychiatry, and each of these schools focuses on a different aspect of the human personality. Each psychiatrist follows whatever system their founding fathers (who often had conflicting views on the causes of mental problems) prescribed.

Psychiatrists from the school of Freud are convinced that most mental disease stems from the suppression of sexual desires and their diagnosis and treatment will be based on this belief. Other psychiatrists, psychologists and psychoanalysts are followers of the many different schools of psychiatry that developed after Freud. Many of them do not believe in Freud's theories any longer, and each of them has its own point of view and treats patients accordingly. Their theories include, for example, the belief that mental problems and disease are the consequence of unconscious conflict stemming from problems with relationships, a wish to escape, inferiority complexes, fear, anxiety and many more. Nobody knows which, if any, of these schools is right, and maybe no one will ever know.

Patients who first of all go to a Jungian psychiatrist and later, if their problems do not improve, go to a psychiatrist who follows the school of, for example, Fromm, will get a completely different diagnosis and treatment without any guarantee that their mental health will improve.

In order to find out what is troubling their patients, psychiatrists usually try to delve into their subconscious minds. The patients usually lie on a couch and talk as much as they feel like. The psychiatrist then tries to put a picture together that fits into their scholastic beliefs.

After I had explained all this to my friend, she followed my advice to consult a physician who specialised in orthomolecular medicine. Three years later the behaviour of her son had improved so much that the child was almost unrecognisable.

Recently I was reading an article in the *Scientific American* about a new theory concerning AD/HD. It suggested that the disorder results from a failure in self-control, when key brain circuits do not develop properly, perhaps because of an altered gene or genes. It is very fashionable to make genes the culprit for anything that goes wrong in the human body or mind. Being a naturopath I always ask 'why' and get to the bottom of a problem. Of course, there are children that are born with genes that cause brain abnormalities, but this would only be the case with a small percentage. There are far too many children with AD/HD and similar disorders, and therefore in most cases the culprits cannot be genes. It seems impossible that suddenly hundreds of thousands of kids have been born with the wrong genes.

The part of the brain that is responsible for self-control consists of many brain cells. If these cells do not get the right fuel, they cannot function normally. Children who lack certain nutrients, because their food does not contain them or their organism cannot assimilate them, usually act in an abnormal way. It has been proved that children often behave in a more normal way when their diet is changed, when their intestines are cleansed and when no more toxins enter their body.

It is interesting that many children do not develop symptoms until late childhood or even early adolescence. This could be due to a slower accumulation of toxic matter in the body. If bad genes had anything to do with it, symptoms would be seen much earlier.

There is very little evidence that child psychiatry really helps and there may even be some dangerous side-effects, mentally as well as physically. With many hours of psychiatric treatment children get into the habit of concentrating far too much on their personal problems. Depending on the personality of the child, this may increase their fears and complexes, or stimulate their ego in the wrong way. It may encourage children to see themselves as very important people with a very interesting disease. In some children this only increases the urge to boast and show off. Others will retreat within themselves even more. With some exceptions, I strongly recommend avoiding consulting a psychiatrist as it may well worsen the problem.

Because of the side-effects of psychiatric drugs like tranquillisers and other mind-altering medication, the danger of a psychiatric consultation is clear. If children have taken one or several drugs that depress the central nervous system or on the contrary accelerate different reactions, there may be psychological side-effects that could have a negative influence on them for the rest of their lives. Such medication may control the condition for which it is prescribed, but usually at great cost. Sometimes the side-effects of a single drug may not be very harmful, but the additional effect of other drugs the child takes or even their interaction with nutritional chemicals might be dangerous.

Of course, there are certain mental and neurological disorders that have their roots in medical intervention or accidents. In such a case psychiatric treatment might be of help, but brain damage is rather rare compared to the great number of children suffering from atypical behaviour. I would certainly not recommend this kind of therapeutic treatment for a child, with the exception of a simple 'talk therapy' whereby children are given the opportunity to talk to a friendly, interested person – and this does not have to be a physician – about their personal problems. Some children do not dare to talk openly to parents, relatives or other people from their own milieu. They would much rather open up to a sympathetic stranger. Troubled children, just like adults, need to talk about their problems.

Physical and mental problems are always interwoven. When children begin to understand the close relationship of body and mind and learn to see their personal problems in a different light, it will not be long before they will try to do something positive to help themselves. We often tend to forget that children with behavioural problems suffer very much. They do not want to hurt people on purpose, but they cannot help what they are doing, as something that is stronger than their willpower is influencing them. Such children would often do anything to be able to behave normally.

Many specialists seem to ignore the living dynamic properties of the brain, viewing it as a simple appliance or a computer. But what about the daily input of molecular substances to the brain? Can improper food-body-brain interactions, sustained by habitual food choices, produce the patterns of dysfunction commonly observed?

AD/HD can be seen as a symptom of a food-driven hypersensitivity disease. This is not a common allergy that can be diagnosed by skin tests. We are talking about delayed patterns of food allergy, or an incompatibility to certain foods, which cannot be detected by those tests.

EMOTIONAL ISSUES

A child may be starved of affection or attention, physical touching, and expressions of caring and love. Parents should try tuning in with their children more often, sharing activities and interests. They should help their children to channel their energy in positive ways, like a good bike ride, skateboarding or outdoor games. This is just as satisfying as running around, yelling and behaving in a crazy way.

Vitamin pills can only help sort out personal problems to a certain extent. However, it always gives the right basis for the right counselling with an interested and very caring therapist; this can really help the child to do the rest. After the biochemical problems are taken care of, the patient is better able to benefit from some counselling, or in very few cases from psychiatric help, if this should really be needed.

Although I usually doubt the value of classical psychiatry for children, there is a new branch of medicine called 'orthomolecular psychiatry'. This could eventually revolutionise medicine; both children and adults are affected by toxic chemicals in food, and a lack of many different nutrients. When will we realise that meddling with the balance of nature is sure to bring about severe consequences?

༄ *Chapter 27* ༄

HOMOEOPATHY

Unlike antibiotics and other strong medicine, homoeopathic remedies have no dangerous side-effects. Homoeopathy uses remedies made from natural substances in very small doses. Homoeopathy is safe for children of all ages, including babies, and also for pregnant women. Future mothers risk the health of their babies when they take any strong medicine. With homoeopathic medicine there is no such risk and these remedies are tested in the only scientific way possible, on normal healthy people. A 'healing remedy' should never have dangerous side-effects.

Strong medication is only acceptable in cases of real emergency. However, this can never heal; it can only suppress the symptoms of a disease.

The homoeopathic approach to attention deficit disorders (ADD and AD/HD) cannot be compared to that of conventional medicine. A homoeopath can choose from over 2,000 different remedies, rather than the small number of conventional medications used to treat ADD and AD/HD. Homoeopathy can offer an effective solution for many children.

Professional homoeopaths will first of all interview children and their parents in detail to discover all their physical, emotional and mental symptoms. Homoeopaths seek to select the substance that would cause similar symptoms when given in an overdose. Then highly diluted, specially prepared doses of that substance are given to the patient. There are about a dozen homoeopathic medicines that might be deemed appropriate for hyperactivity, aggression or autism.

Homoeopathy helps millions of people all over the world and has been used by the British royal family for many generations. Not only physical, but also most mental diseases and problems can be treated with homoeopathic remedies. As homoeopathic medicine is so suitable for children, more and more paediatricians prescribe it for their patients. Homoeopathic pills are sweet, so children like to take them and make no fuss about it. Homoeopathy can be said to be definitely effective in treating the emotional disorders that commonly occur in the children of the twenty-first century.

At the moment there are over 2,000 different homoeopathic remedies and each remedy corresponds with special symptoms of disease, with character traits and mental problems. A homoeopath has to study for many years, often longer than any other physician has to study. Homoeopathic medicine is not only a special kind of medicine, it is also an art.

The first time homoeopaths see patients, the consultation may take up to two or three hours and they may ask hundreds of questions. When treating babies or small children the parents will be asked these questions instead, and the homoeopath will observe the reactions of the child at the same time. In classical homoeopathy there always is one optimal remedy for each child that exactly fits. It is extremely difficult to find this remedy and the doctor will have to study every detail of the character, the behaviour and the physical health of the child very thoroughly. Luckily, there still are some gifted homoeopaths that can find this remedy – if not right away, then some time in the near future.

This special remedy has to do with what is called the 'miasma' of the child. The miasma is the sum total of the consequences of inherited physical, mental, emotional and spiritual foundations of the child. These may have been influenced by the physical and mental condition of the mother during pregnancy, by vaccine damage, or by environmental and emotional stress in early life.

There are many things that can harm the unborn child and the little baby. Babies are extremely sensitive to loud noises, hard voices, discordant modern music, or a lack of love and attention. They need a harmonious atmosphere, soft natural light, and love and care during the daytime, as well as peace and tranquillity at night.

Unfortunately, many babies and small children do not get much of those things nowadays, and there is too much stress, which impedes the optimal development of the child. Besides these mental and emotional causes, there are also different physical influences that can destroy the healthy equilibrium in a child and the most important one is the wrong nutrition.

I hope that God protects little children who are bombarded when ill with strong medicine in order to suppress the symptoms. If the excretion of toxins by way of the skin is suppressed, the organism will look for another way to excrete those toxins and that may be recurrent colds, ear infections, bronchitis, asthma and so on. The child will be 'treated' for these diseases and in the process the pathways by which toxins can leave the body will be closed. Again the organism has to find a new escape route for the accumulating toxic substances. All the emergency measures the organism tries to take will be pounced on right away and in this way small children can fall into a vicious circle in which they may be trapped for the rest of their lives. After a while some of these reactions, like colds, ear infections or asthma, may become chronic and the more medication the child is given, the more serious the resulting health problems will be.

A child who has intelligent parents is very lucky. They may take their baby to a good homoeopath or naturopath and with the help of a special diet, with homoeopathic medicine, herbs, water treatments and other natural healing methods, many problems can be solved. The sooner a child is treated in a natural way, the sooner it will be healthy and happy.

There are two different schools of homoeopathy. The first and oldest one is, as I explained, the school that treats a patient with only one kind of remedy at the time, corresponding to their miasma. If a small quantity of the right remedy is given, even only once or twice, the whole personality of a patient can change within one or two weeks. With small children especially this is an amazing occurrence and people who have never seen it happen before can hardly believe it.

However, sometimes it is important to eliminate the worst symptoms quickly. This might be, for example, a very painful earache, a nose that is dripping constantly or swollen tonsils. In that case some homoeopathic physicians may decide first to give a homoeopathic mixture. Some homoeopaths do not like using these, because the mixtures are not directed at the miasma of the patient. However, although these mixed homoeopathic formulas only have a suppressive function and resemble allopathic (conventional) treatment in that way, they do not harm the patient. Many such mixed remedies show excellent results, and in my opinion it is very important to help a suffering child right away. Later there is plenty of time to find the exact homoeopathic formula for the child.

Only the right classical homoeopathic remedy can really be a cure and in the long run, properly selected homoeopathic medicine can be a great help for many children. Often only a few doses of the right remedy are needed and sometimes just one dose does the trick.

Here are some homoeopathic remedies that might help your child in case of sleeplessness, hyperactivity, aggressiveness, fears, timidity, tantrums, and all the other problems mentioned in this book.

Chamomilla
Stramonium
Cina
Hyoscyamos niger
Arsenicum
Argenticum nitricum
Tarantula hispanica
Veratrum album
Calcarea phosphoricum
Kalibromatum
Lycopodium
Medorrhinum

Chamomilla is often used for small babies to help with sleeping problems and restlessness. Later it also helps with teething problems. As soon as a chamomilla child has attracted attention, it stops being fidgety. These children may become overtired because of their own restlessness and start crying. Do not give chamomile tea when the child is taking chamomilla as a homoeopathic remedy, as they will cancel each other out.

Stramonium should be used for temper, extreme fear, tantrums, stress, uncontrollable aggression and violence. The child may stammer and suffer from convulsions, and possibly sleepwalk. These children often talk in such a way that nobody understands what they really mean; their speech is loud, fast and incoherent. Stramonium is for children with severe hyperactivity and possible violent agitation.

Cina helps children that are physically aggressive and even as babies try to bite their mother or their siblings.

Hyoscyamos niger is often right for children that have maniac or sexualised symptoms.

Arsenicum children are restless all the time and seem to be driven. They are frightened and do not have any courage when the environment changes or new people come into their lives. They hate being alone. They can also be quite fussy. These little children are the ones that turn their heads away from strangers. As they expend so much energy all the time, they soon become exhausted and often have an interrupted sleep. They are hypersensitive and hate noise. They easily get colds and headaches. These children usually have great problems with the digestion of milk products, sugar and wheat.

Tarantula hispanica children love lively music, dancing and bright colours; they are always terribly restless, stressed and in a hurry. They like tapping and drumming. Grown-up tarantula patients may have a tendency for kleptomania and may also tell lies. They may talk too much, they may have a tendency for kleptomania, but they often have a heart of gold. Tarantula people may break anything that comes into their hands, and grind their teeth. Their muscles are often twitching and jerking.

Argenticum nitricum is indicated for children who are always in a hurry and worry all the time. They cannot concentrate and often try to explain themselves. Their physical development is usually pretty fast. They love sweets, but these influence their behaviour, as they cannot digest them. They frequently get tummy-aches, conjunctivitis or tonsillitis, and they often have skin problems and itching, and suffer when the weather is very warm. These children are usually thin. They hate crowds and love to be outdoors.

Veratrum album children can be very affectionate, especially girls, who may be kissing people all the time. Although some of these children are often extremely restless, their actions may become almost ritualistic and they cannot stop when doing something they are interested in. They may rush around and change their occupation all the time. They may be nail-biters. As babies they may suffer from ear infections, diarrhoea and perspiration.

Calcarea phosphoricum children are restless devils who like to play tricks. They often have enlarged tonsils, suffer from gas and have swollen tummies.

Kalibromatum children are always doing something with their hands. They are never still. If no toy is at hand, they crack their knuckles.

Lycopodium children are more tired or restless in the afternoon. Even when they are very tired, they never keep still. They are usually very intelligent and are easily bored if something is not interesting enough for them. They often look older than their years.

Medorrhinum children are irritable and in a hurry, and often become very agitated. Medorrhinum babies often suffer from nappy rashes and other skin problems. Bronchitis and asthma also often occur.

Properly selected and administered homoeopathic medicine can be a godsend for hyperactive children. It can help them slow down, relax and feel more internally secure. Homoeopathy can also strengthen their constitution so that they feel stronger and less ill.

Self-treatment with homoeopathic remedies can be beneficial for short-term problems. For a more permanent solution to a chronic condition such as hyperactivity, however, it is important to consult a qualified homoeopathic practitioner. One dose of the proper remedy will usually last six months to a year or more, and the treatment will not have to be repeated unless the child's behaviour deteriorates. If a youngster is on stimulant medication, the homoeopathic medicine may need to be given more often. About

70 per cent of children professionally treated with homoeopathy for hyperactivity improve significantly, and many of them improve dramatically.

The beauty of the action of homoeopathic drops and remedies is that they function as a catalyst for the body's own inner healing mechanisms and resources to go into action to correct health imbalances. If the remedy taken is unnecessary, nothing happens! If not used excessively, there are no harmful side-effects to worry about with homoeopathy, unlike most prescription drugs.

❧ Chapter 28 ❧

HELPING WITH HERBS

Herbs have been used for thousands of years for physical, mental and emotional problems. They have no side-effects and are widely available.

Herbs are often used in their most natural form as herbal teas, or they are made up into capsules, tablets or liquidised. As tea or drops they are often used for the treatment of hyperactive, tired, over-stressed, frightened or mentally disturbed children. They also help with physical problems.

Maybe the best-known herbal remedy is valerian. This herb has a very relaxing effect on the central nervous system. It is not habit-forming.

Red clover is a blood purifier and is often used as a tea. It also has a relaxing effect when it is used over a longer period of time. To make tea take one tablespoon to a cup of water; steep for about 15 minutes and drink half a cup in the morning and at night.

Chamomile tea is a wonderful relaxant for babies and small children and when drunk before bedtime helps children to sleep. There is no need to sweeten it, as small children like the natural taste of this herb, and it is important not to give your children a taste for sweetened drinks.

Lime blossom is also relaxing, but a little stronger than chamomile.

Catnip is often used if a child does not sleep well. It is safe and very relaxing.

California poppy is a safe sedative for hyperactive and aggressive children. Usually it is mixed with other herbs. It also helps children to sleep better.

Wild lettuce is another well-known herbal remedy. It is often contained in a mixture of other different herbs. It is a sedative and a sleeping aid.

Lemon balm is a nice herb that tastes like lemon and has relaxing properties. Good for insomnia.

Skullcap calms the mind and is a relaxant. Give your child one dose three times a week, for three months. Do not give it to children under six years of age.

Avena (wild oats) calms the nerves. Give your child one dose daily for one month.

Other relaxing and safe herbs are: passion flower, liquorice, fennel, berries, linden blossom, milk thistle, melissa officinales, Irish moss, gotu kola, hops, evening primrose and kava-kava.

Kelp and nettle tea help cleanse the body of heavy-metal poisoning.

Eleuthero helps with depression and corrects blood sugar metabolism and adrenal function.

Evening primrose oil, 2–3 grams daily, is being recommended by the Hyperactive Children's Support Group of Great Britain. It corrects the essential fatty acid deficiency noted in some AD/HD children.

Certain botanical scents may calm a hyperactive child. Mix one drop each of rosemary, sage, lavender and chamomile oil in one-eighth of a cup of olive oil, and use this aromatic oil to rub your child's feet and spine at bedtime.

ALTERNATIVE TREATS FOR HYPERACTIVE CHILDREN

Instead of soft drinks (many of which are loaded with sugar) or bottled fruit juice, which contains a considerable amount of fructose, there are a number of delicious herbal teas that can be sweetened with stevia or liquorice. Herbal teas such as chamomile, peppermint, spearmint, orange peel, cinnamon and hibiscus sweetened with stevia or liquorice are especially nice.

Here is a recipe for a healthy soft drink:

Hibiscus Cooler
Hibiscus 3 parts
Orange peel 1 part
Cinnamon 1 part
Blend together and before serving add a small handful of
fresh spearmint or peppermint leaves. Sweeten with apple
juice (1 part juice to 4 parts tea) or use stevia.

Celery and lettuce have a calming effect on the nerves. Try celery
stuffed with peanut (or other nut) butter.

Most herbs that herbalists (or phytotherapists, specialists in
herbs) recommend for hyperactivity are widely available in natural
food stores as single herbs or included in formulas. They are sold as
herb teas, or as finished products like capsules, tablets or liquid
extracts (tinctures).

Parents can benefit from the above as well, since they would also
be exhausted and under stress with a hyperactive child.
Phytotherapists do not only help children; they can also help their
parents.

Herbal therapy should be always included in a broad treatment
plan, together with diet, counselling and other treatments
mentioned in this book.

Chapter 29

ORTHOMOLECULAR MEDICINE

Although many physicians do not yet even know the meaning of the word, at last orthomolecular medicine has been recognised as a unique healing method and has emerged at the cutting edge of mainstream medicine. Recently orthomolecular medicine has become so well known that physicians from all over the world attend conventions on the subject.

Orthomolecular psychiatry is a very interesting development that could eventually revolutionise medicine itself, for it is not only children that are affected by toxic chemicals in our food, and a lack of nutrients. Although hardly anybody seems to realise it, most adults also have mental and behavioural problems. Unfortunately, most of our political and financial leaders suffer from the same problems as our children, and it is mainly because of this that there is no peace and security in the world any more. It is high time we realised that biochemical malfunctioning of the brain and the nervous system is at the root of many political decisions that may change our world forever.

Orthomolecular medicine evolved over time into a discipline under the direction of Linus Pauling, winner of two Nobel prizes, in 1968. It is designed to enable individuals to achieve optimum health by utilising only naturally occurring substances (e.g. vitamins, minerals, enzymes, trace elements and co-enzymes). The proper balance of these substances in the body is the key to reaching physical, mental and emotional health and stability.

Orthomolecular medicine looks for biochemical rather than

psychological causes of disorders. The doctrine believes that the human body is like a biochemical factory, and when it does not receive enough raw materials (nutrients) or receives toxins, malfunctioning results. The brain becomes biochemically disordered and views the world abnormally; other people suddenly appear peculiar in their behaviour and motives. Only when the brain receives the right nutrients do these misapprehensions disappear. Over time it has been discovered that malnutrition brought on by the consumption of refined and processed foods such as the ever-popular white bread can initiate disease and psychiatric problems. Suddenly, it became obvious that a person's diet was fundamental in determining the future health of an individual.

Many conservative physicians and nutritionists are generally opposed to orthomolecular treatment. Having helped set the government's official nutrition standards, they naturally resist the notion that our national diet could cause any vitamin deficiencies that might lead to mental and emotional problems.

Brain cells need more than 30 per cent of all the nutrients we consume and if there is a lack of some of these nutrients, they cannot function in an optimal way. Many diseases that were considered as recently as half a century ago to be caused solely by a malfunctioning of the brain, and therefore in most cases incurable, can now be treated and often cured.

Peter B. Breggin wrote in his excellent book, *Toxic Psychiatry*:

> A child's state of health is his state of nutrition. When minerals, vitamins, amino acids, enzymes or even hormones are deficient in a child's system, the result can be a disturbed biochemical balance that causes impaired functions in his brain. Orthomolecular therapy means supplying the cells with the right mixture of nutrients. Adjusting the diet, eliminating junk foods and ingesting the proper doses of essential nutrients, can correct the chemical imbalances.

He also said that 'hyperactivity is the most frequent justification for drugging children'.

Besides a lack of nutrients, an avalanche of toxic substances in our food and environment hinder the normal functioning and chemical balance of our brain and nervous system. Children especially react within a short time when certain important nutrients such as vitamins, minerals, amino acids, enzymes and hormones are missing. All children are different and they all react in their own way when important nutrients are missing. There are children who have very special nutritional requirements, for example of certain vitamins, and they can only be helped if these needs are discovered and taken care of. In stressful situations the body uses up far more nutrients than in normal times. Stress can occur when children are very sensitive, afraid or angry, when they have too much homework and cannot relax, when, especially in winter, classrooms are illuminated exclusively by artificial light, and so on.

However, if the organism of a child receives plenty of nutrients, problems are much easier to overcome and life becomes simpler. Practitioners of orthomolecular medicine are dedicated to the task of finding out what nutrients are missing in their patients. Every individual is a unique biochemical creature and this principle is at the core of the discipline.

Many people suffer from food allergies or incompatibilities, and often toxins cause different health problems and diseases. Therefore, orthomolecular physicians use special methods of investigation and examination. At the same time they are in favour of the kind of psychological support that can be given by counselling. They try to remove as many toxins as possible from the body and to supply the cells with the right combination of nutrients. They emphasise the necessity of sound nutrition and prescribe mega-vitamin treatment if it is needed. Although orthomolecular medicine also treats disorders such as allergies, asthma, chronic fatigue, depression, diabetes, menopause, heart disease and osteoporosis, the treatment is famous mainly for its success in helping patients with schizophrenia, attention deficit disorder, hyperactivity, autism and other mental problems and diseases.

As yet, few parents realise that they are ruining the health of their children by permitting them to eat junk food, crisps and all kinds of coloured sweets, as well as letting them drink Coca-Cola and similar beverages. The parents themselves are often the victims when their children become unmanageable, aggressive and nasty, have learning and behaviour problems, or suffer from ear infections, respiratory difficulties or sleeplessness and many other problems. Many parents do not realise that by simply changing the eating and drinking habits of their children and giving them the mega-vitamin and mineral doses that orthomolecular physicians prescribe, such weak, pale, sick and badly behaving children can often, within a few weeks or months, become happy, healthy and normal. For many young patients, orthomolecular medicine is a real godsend and I hope that in the future many more physicians will specialise in it, and be able to give help without risking harmful side-effects.

It cannot be denied that some mental disorders can be triggered by stress, sudden shock or trauma, or an accumulation of disappointments and frustrations that make life too much to bear. However, practitioners of orthomolecular psychiatry are convinced that the most important causative factor is biochemical.

❧ *Chapter 30* ❧

THE IMPORTANCE OF LIGHT

For thousands of years people have revered the sun as a great healer and it is easy to understand why some cultures worshipped it. We are creatures of light. Health is not possible for us without it. After being in the sun we always feel happier and healthier, and we have more energy. We are not just imagining this; sunlight really improves our health.

Newbold, the author of *Mega-Nutrients for Your Nerves*, writes: 'Before we began civilising ourselves into semi-invalidism, we received an abundance of full-spectrum light, the kind of light that nature provides for us in the form of sunlight.' Sunlight, along with food, air and water, is the most important survival factor of human life.

The study of light as a health-promoting factor has received far too little attention. Although a great number of books have been written on the subject, the general practitioner knows very little about the importance of light. Also, most physicians do not realise that many health problems of our time are at least partly due to a lack of pure natural light.

The light that several scientists consider a 'super-nutrient' is full-spectrum light, which comes from the sun. Light bulbs of a special design that simulate sunlight have been available for a few decades. Bulbs of exactly the same spectrum quality as sunlight have not yet been designed, but lighting with such bulbs is still much better than the kind of lighting most of us we have in our homes, schools and workplaces.

Fluorescent light is disastrous for our health, as it weakens our muscle strength and mental activity and happens to be the most nutrient deficient of all lightening devices. Even ordinary light bulbs are preferable to the total artificiality of the fluorescent environment. John Ott, of Sarasota, Florida, a pioneer of light and health research, has been warning for the last 50 years of the unhealthy effects of some kinds of light. Lately much basic research has been done that supports his ideas.

Russian scientists have been studying the health effects of various kinds of light for many decades and applying their knowledge in factories and schools there. They have proved that full-spectrum lighting improves industrial production, helps academic performance in schools and even increases the tolerance to environmental pollutants. Such light has a positive influence on the behaviour of students and lessens fatigue. Germany and other European countries have researched this, and found that the lighting normally used in schools can make children irritable, restless, nervous and hyperactive, and they may suffer from headaches, eyestrain, stress and fatigue, and from viral and cold infections. In some schools where the usual lighting was replaced by full-spectrum lighting, within a few weeks the children became more relaxed and friendly, and their academic performance and behaviour improved.

We all know that vitamin D is synthesised by ultraviolet rays. Vitamin D facilitates the absorption of calcium and a lack of sunlight can result in nutritional deficiencies. Most enzymes, hormones and vitamins need light for proper functioning. Studies have shown that different forms of light stimulate various enzymatic reactions in the human body. It is a known fact that full-spectrum light has specific assignments concerning our physical and mental health. Light entering our eyes is converted into nerve impulses that influence the most important brain centres, like the hypothalamus, which secretes hormones that stimulate or suppress the release of hormones in the pituitary and pineal glands, which control the entire endocrine system.

However, light enters not only by way of the eyes, but also through our skin and cranial bones. Rays of full-spectrum light stimulate the pineal gland, a small gland in the head, directly. This gland secretes melatonin, a hormone that controls many physical and mental functions. It is easy to understand, therefore, that full-spectrum light can be of great help in treating many diseases and mental problems.

Today many children suffer from a lack of exposure to natural sunlight. In their homes, schools or day-care centres the indoor lighting is sometimes so poor that it actually destroys the defence mechanisms of the body and causes physical as well as mental problems. A study of three American school districts suggests that one good way to raise test scores is to let the sunshine in. Investigators found that students exposed to the most daylight had significantly higher test scores. In Seattle, students in light-filled schools scored 9–13 per cent higher in maths and reading tests than those with the least light.

It is not only humans that are weakened by bad lighting – any animal or plant deprived of light will lose its strength after a while, and perish. It is not sufficient to take your child on a holiday for a few weeks each year; children need fresh air and full-spectrum light whenever possible. In exchange for the comforts of modern life, we have imprisoned ourselves between walls and in towns, where fresh air and sunlight are often a luxury. It is high time to do something about it, and municipalities should realise that in future building more parks and free space should have absolute priority, first of all for the health of our children.

WHAT YOU CAN DO

Take your children outside the city as often as possible. You do not have to go to faraway places on holiday; the most important thing is that children come into contact with nature. They need to be able to play and run in the sunshine and fresh air. In winter, you could rent a light box for home use and let any member of the family who feels low sit in front of it for several hours a day. Children can play and adults can read while doing this. In Switzerland, in the town of Basel, I observed about 30 female patients who were being treated for serious depression in a big hospital. These women sat in front a wall which was covered with full-spectrum lighting devices. They sat there for hours each day knitting and talking and having a wonderful time, while being cured of their depression, and sometimes also of migraine headaches.

Change the lighting in your house. The quantity of light is not half as important as the quality. If it is available and you can afford it, buy full-spectrum light bulbs or install full-spectrum lighting in your home. Last but not least, convince your MPs, schoolteachers and other influential people that good lighting in all buildings is of the utmost importance.

🌺 Chapter 31 🌺

FOOD AND CRIMINAL BEHAVIOUR

Youth criminality in Great Britain recently went up by 49 per cent – in 2001, just one year! It seems incredible that this can happen in our own country. Every one of us is concerned with the problem of increasing violence in our affluent society and we all wonder how it has become so bad.

Of course, there have always been criminals and crime, but this new development is very alarming and many people do not feel safe any more. Formerly, most of the time law-breakers had a personal and often understandable reason to burgle, or even murder someone – it may have been a crime of passion, because they were broke and could not feed their family, or other simple reasons. Such crimes were hardly ever committed by normal, hard-working citizens, as they were far too busy earning a living.

Many people are of the opinion that the youth of today is under the devastating influence of crime programmes on television, video games, bad company, working parents who are seldom at home, lack of education and drugs. Of course, the old reasons for committing crimes still exist as well. All these causes of crime are valid, and can increase problems up to a certain point, but without doubt there is more to it than that.

Lately there has been a completely new and very frightening development. Nowadays it often happens that when young people who murder, commit arson or mug old people are asked why they did it say that they really do not know. It seems that while doing those things, they act like zombies, under a kind of compulsion. We know that everything that is happening in the world at a certain time is always connected to other developments. Nothing that happens stands out as a single event, separated from the rest of the world. As soon as anything in our world alters, everything connected to it starts adapting itself to the change, although it sometimes means a turn for the worse.

During the last century nothing changed as much as the environment, and people have also changed in many ways. Man-made toxins have invaded our environment, our bodies and our minds. We tried, with the help of new toxins, to eradicate all disease and at first we seemed to succeed, but soon we were confronted with a flood of new, formerly unknown chronic diseases that did not respond any more to treatment with antibiotics or other toxins. Medicine has reached a dead-end street. Because we were so busy trying to cure the diseases of the body, we almost forgot to do something about diseases of the mind.

Not only our body, but also our mind has been infiltrated on all levels with thousands of different toxins, through our skin, our lungs and our food. As our most intimate contact with our environment is through the food we eat, most toxic matter comes into our body in this way. Everything entering the body that cannot be changed into endogenic material (substances that are like the body's own matter) and used is recognised as dangerous by the organism and triggers off defensive reactions. Never in the history of humankind have so many foreign and dangerous substances entered the body, and defensive reactions against these toxins cost us an enormous amount of energy and ruin our health.

Our brain needs about one-third of all nutrients we assimilate or produce. When the diet of a child is lacking from conception onwards in many essential nutrients or contains an excess of toxins, the body as well as the brain will be in bad shape. Such infants will cry much more than healthy infants do and when feeling low, teenagers or adults will often go on a binge and consume nothing but sugar-laden foods or drinks. When teenagers have a nutrition-poor diet, this negative pattern escalates. Other dangerous crutches are coffee, beer, wine, strong alcohol and ultimately addictive harmful drugs.

On the Internet I found a very interesting overall view of the annual consumption of low-nutrient food, concerning American teenagers and adolescents:

> Doughnuts (number) 756
> Cakes and cookies (pounds) 60
> Ice cream (gallons) 23
> Potato chips (pounds) 7
> Candy (pounds) 22
> Gum (sticks) 200
> Soda pop (servings) 365
> Fat (pounds) 90
> Refined sugar (pounds) 134

Besides this, an enormous amount of toxic additives, artificial flavourings or colourings are added to most of our food, especially to junk food. A poor lifestyle inevitably leads to bad behaviour and often to criminal activities necessary for obtaining expensive drugs.

Because all these foods bring no vitamins, minerals or other nutrients, the body must use storage supplies to feed the brain, and many times those supplies are not available. Therefore the area of the brain which controls thought, learning and behaviour shuts down and converts all the energy available to the areas of the brain that are needed for the survival of the race, like the areas for food, sex and the fight-or-flight syndrome.

There is a ten-fold variation in individual requirements for certain nutrients, such as vitamins and minerals. Stressed teenagers and adults on a highly refined diet require still-higher levels to maintain a normal metabolism. Most vitamins affect brain chemistry to some degree and if chronically increased requirements are not met, abnormal brain chemistry may develop. Vitamin B3 (nicotinamide), folic acid and ascorbic acid (vitamin C) are especially important for normal brain functions.

It has been proved that often a criminal mind can be linked to bad nutritional habits and some specific foods. Psychiatrists in New York found almost 50 years ago that many criminals lived almost exclusively on junk food and soft drinks. The fast food they ate was usually cooked in oil that had been reheated many times. When oil is reheated it often develops certain toxic substances that enter the brain through the bloodstream. Old, rancid oil is not only a vitamin and mineral robber; it can also damage and paralyse brain or nerve cells. Many criminals act as if they are in a kind of trance, and do not really know what is going on. It is quite interesting that some hyperactive children can behave in a similar way. Of course, oil is not the only culprit, but in combination with other refined and unnatural foods its regular consumption can have serious consequences, not only for the body but also for the mind.

Sugar replaces calories from healthy food; as a consequence there are deficiencies. Sugary foods tend to contain high levels of chemical dyes and preservatives, and these substances might stimulate anti-social behaviour.

The life of teenagers is full of stress and noise. An episode of severe stress is often the trigger of a mental breakdown. This is because during stressful situations we require higher levels of certain vitamins and minerals than normally. If this requirement comes on top of a generally poor vitamin–mineral status, combined with an inadequate diet, the brain just does not receive enough nutrients to function in a normal way. All this may incapacitate the brain.

Dr William Walsh, who gave a lecture at the last convention of orthomolecular physicians in Vancouver, often did volunteer work for a prisoner assistance programme for convicts and ex-offenders at a prison in Illinois. There he became aware of the interesting phenomenon, that some of the most violent and incorrigible prisoners seemed to have come from good stable families and had siblings who had turned out to be good citizens. Walsh began to wonder why siblings in the same families could turn out so differently. He came to the conclusion that the bad behaviour of many teenagers was not the result of an unhappy family life or a bad upbringing. In his opinion, it was due to an innate or acquired biochemical disposition. Walsh founded the non-profit-making Health Research Institute with the intent of studying the possible biochemical links with behaviour. Later Walsh met the late Carl Pfeiffer, a pioneer in orthomolecular research, who suggested that Walsh would do well to examine trace elements – particularly copper and zinc – as a cause of behaviour disorders. Walsh's group then conducted many experiments to determine the biochemical profiles of delinquent adolescents, hardened criminals and even serial killers. They discovered that behavioural syndromes were strongly correlated with four biochemical profiles, distinct enough to distinguish violence-prone individuals *simply by looking at their lab results*. It was found that many criminals have high levels of copper and low levels of zinc compared to non-violent people. Cadmium and lead prevent the absorption of zinc. Too much sugar and alcohol also reduce zinc absorption. Dr Walsh was not the only physician interested in this kind of research. On the Internet one can find hundreds of samples of such research and most of them confirm Walsh's findings.

Searching for solutions to prison violence, in the spring of 1981 the Los Angeles County Board of Supervisors held hearings on the alleged link between diet and human behaviour. The board was so convinced by testimony about the sugar–violence link that they ordered the replacement of all soft drinks and junk food snacks in the prison with fruit juices and health foods. High-sugar desserts and cereals were also banned and as a consequence the behaviour of the criminals improved considerably. After only three months of the new diet, anti-social behaviour among all inmates fell by 44 per cent and remained low thereafter.

In many jails and correction facilities such experiments were highly successful, but until recently mainstream medicine took little notice. This is a great pity as the number of criminal offences could be reduced, many thousands of criminals rehabilitated and terrible crimes prevented.

It would also be worthwhile to change the eating and living habits of the younger generation in order to prevent the development of AD/HD. The behaviour complex of AD/HD often has lifelong implications, as the personality of the child forms around the dysfunctional patterns. With persisting illness and failure, low self-esteem, social maladjustment and anti-social behaviour develop. Unpleasant, hostile behaviour in the younger child grows into delinquent patterns in early adolescence, and later, anti-social or criminal behaviour if uncorrected. Hyperactivity in children often leads to juvenile delinquency, as well as criminal behaviour in adults.

Because of poor eating habits whereby high amounts of refined carbohydrates are eaten (see the chapter about low blood sugar), many children, teenagers and adults suffer from erratic blood sugar levels. Sometimes their blood sugar level is high (hyperglycaemia) and at other times far too low (hypoglycaemia). Those who are hypoglycaemic have an erratic blood sugar level after ingesting sweet foods. Emotions closely follow the blood sugar level and often go up and down in quick succession. In children this may produce bouts of hyperactivity followed by exhaustion, and in adults violence and all kinds of neuroses. In mentally unstable individuals it may trigger a manic episode of great, uncontrollable excitement and violence. During a period of hyperglycaemia too much energy is being generated by the brain, which may lead to mental agitation, irritability or uncontrollable excitement. When the burst of energy has passed, there is a lack of energy and this may lead to a lethargic, listless or depressed condition, in some cases even suicide.

Allergic responses to refined carbohydrates and other foods have been known to reduce the levels of neurotransmitters (small messenger molecules) in our brains. When these are in short supply in the brain, behaviour can be affected. Small molecules such as artificial food colours or salicylates can be carried from the intestine to the brain through the bloodstream. In the brain, these molecules interfere with the chemical and electrical functioning of our brain cells. The effects can also be produced by drugs, cosmetics, food additives and preservatives, and it takes very little of the offending chemical to produce the toxic effect.

According to the National Institute of Mental Health, 6.4 million Americans are under some form of mental health care and an estimated 10 per cent of all Americans are in need of such care. That translates into over 20 million people. The possibility that mental illness can be brought under control and that the number of criminal offences could be greatly reduced by correcting nutritional deficiencies is a significant discovery and we still have not given up hope that one day governmental and medical authorities will realise this.

Chapter 32

CLEANSING THE ORGANISM, DETOXIFYING THE BODY

If you read my book *Healing in the 21st Century* you will probably remember what I wrote in the introduction. For those who did not read the book, I will briefly explain why cleansing the body of waste products and toxins is at least as important as eating the right food.

Toxins are produced inside the body as waste materials from dead cells, dead bacteria and other sources. Other toxins come from food, drink, polluted water and air. Within a short time, toxins in our body combine with enzymes, destroy them and cause havoc. They impair metabolic functions and the lack of enzymes results in a reduced capacity to assimilate important nutrients that are necessary for a healthy body and mind.

These metabolic disorders may originate right after birth or even before birth, because of the future mother's bad diet and lifestyle. As a consequence the child may become hyperactive or suffer from other behavioural and mental problems.

While working in your kitchen you would never put some fresh food into a container with spoiled food, as in that case the fresh food would also spoil in no time. The same goes for the intestinal tract. It is often a waste of time and money to buy and prepare healthy food for children when their intestines are filled with waste products and toxins. If their intestines are not clean, children cannot assimilate the healthy food you prepare for them.

When people eat simple and wholesome food, everything goes according to plan. The intestine has a built-in cleansing mechanism that works quite well as long as one is reasonably healthy. However, when too many sweets, chocolate or junk food are eaten, the organism cannot cope and digestion stagnates. More and more food particles that cannot be digested accumulate in the intestinal tract and start fermenting and spoiling. But that is not all. You probably know that during the nutrient exchange from the intestines to the blood, the digested food has to pass through little holes in the intestinal wall, through a kind of filter system. Modern food often contains very sharp and aggressive chemicals that clog up or even damage part of this system.

As a consequence some valuable nutrients cannot enter the blood. On the other hand, all kinds of toxins may enter the portal vein, the big blood vessel that takes the blood to the liver. Too many toxins flood the entire body with all its organs, tissues and body cells and the organism needs to expend an enormous amount of energy in order to neutralise and to fight all these toxins.

When the liver, which is our main detoxification organ, becomes overloaded, it cannot cope and toxins will be stored in many places in the body: in fat cells, brain cells, heart cells and even in the bones. No wonder our children are often tired and very nervous.

Because of all this, it is advisable that before doing anything else the organism of your child should be cleansed. If the body is clean and no more toxins enter by way of the daily food, there is a good chance that after some time the health of your child will improve.

First of all the accumulation of waste materials in the intestines must be disposed of. Even young children may already suffer from constipation. Their bowels may not move regularly and sometimes so much waste has accumulated that it has become a compact mass that sticks to the walls of the intestines. Even children who go to the toilet regularly may have this problem, as each day just a little bit of undigestible toxic substances stay against the walls of the intestines and accumulate there. Do not give your child any strong laxatives. The best way to clean the intestines is an enema with lukewarm water or chamomile tea. When children are small, you will have to do this very carefully and after taking professional advice. Always involve them in your actions and explain to them what you are doing and why. Bigger children can do this themselves.

To boys you should explain that inside cleanliness is very important for the development of the muscles and you could tell girls that they will be more attractive when their insides are clean. Many children get acne or pimples when their intestines are filled with toxins.

Once the intestines are cleansed (in the beginning you may have to do this daily and later perhaps once a week), you can start on a detoxifying programme for the rest of the body.

Always remember that this is only worthwhile when no more junk food is eaten and as few toxins as possible enter the body. There are many herbs and herb teas available in health-food shops that have cleansing properties for the liver and other organs. The smaller a child, the weaker the concentration of the herbal treatment should be. Never treat a small child with strong medication.

Many homoeopathic remedies also have excellent cleansing properties. Which remedy has to be used depends on many things, like the personality of the child and the miasma in the case of classical homoeopathy. Outside sports and walking in the fresh air are a wonderful aid to detoxifying the body. Swimming is excellent. Sweating cleanses the entire organism and brushing or rubbing the skin helps to clear the lymphatic system.

By eating the right food and drinking only water or herbal teas the blood will be cleansed automatically.

❧ Chapter 33 ❧

STRESS, ADDICTION AND DRUGS

Evidence is growing that stress lies at the core of most physical, mental and social problems of our time. Stress is a part of life. We all need a certain amount of stress in order to improve and develop our mental and physical potentials. The right amount of stress can be a challenge; life without stress would be extremely dull. However, in our time we suffer from far too much stress. There is too much noise, and there are too many people and far too many toxins in our food, in the water, in the soil and in the air around us. Also, the aggressive and egotistical behaviour of many people towards their fellow human beings is a very serious cause of stress. When it is of long duration, this kind of stress can cause not only physical diseases, like high blood pressure and gastric and duodenal ulcers, but also various kinds of mental problems and diseases.

First we should know what stress really is. Stress is a normal reaction to changes in our daily life. Stress can be physical, mental or both, and as long as a particular form of stress does not last too long, it can be a positive experience.

From the earliest beginnings, human life was often endangered and adrenaline made people aware of these dangers and prepared the body, as well as the mind for possible flight or fight. These reactions are still the same today, even when the stress exists only in our imagination.

Hans Selye, a Canadian physician, noticed that in the early stages of different infectious diseases, or when injected with a toxic substance, his patients always exhibited the same kind of symptoms. Mental traumas set off similar reactions, following the same sequence. First there is an alarm reaction, whereby important hormonal changes take place. As a result of these changes the adrenal glands become enlarged, the lymph nodes and other white blood cell-producing organs swell up and then shrink, and bleeding appears in the stomach and the intestines. In this way the human body prepares itself for defensive actions. If the stress is not severe and lasts only for a short time, everything soon returns to normal and the patient recovers quickly.

Medical doctors, and especially naturopaths, know that such a short reaction can immunise patients against future attacks of the same kind of toxin or 'stressor'. Next time their reactions to the same kind of stress will be less severe and the defensive capabilities of the organism will have increased. Similar reactions take place in case of mental stress.

However, when the stress is more severe and lasts for a longer time, the second stage begins and we try to adapt to the new situation, assuming that we can resist the effects of stress indefinitely. Therein lies the danger. Believing that we are immune to the effects of stress, we typically fail to do anything about it.

In the third stage, exhaustion begins and our self-defence mechanisms cannot cope with the stressor any more. By and by the stress-fighting reserves succumb and finally the whole organism breaks down. At this point serious physical and mental diseases may develop.

By learning relaxation and stress-management techniques, it is possible to improve your overall health and change many negative destructive thoughts into positive healing reactions.

Dr Selye also made the observation that the hormonal changes which take place as soon as a person is confronted with a stressful situation are due, at least partly, to the chemical make-up of each individual. He was convinced that during stress the body loses its chemical balance and could be put right by chemical intervention.

Although many scientists did not agree with his ideas, pharmaceutical companies smelled big business and billions of dollars were and are still being made selling mind-changing medication. However, such medication often does more harm than good, because when stress is suppressed by the use of strong medication many patients lose their former personality and become like vegetables. Always in a hurry to suppress symptoms and make money, the pharmaceutical industry and the medical establishment ignored one of the most important natural laws. This law, which predominates in all natural processes, decrees that only the weakest stimuli can restore health and well-being, that stronger stimuli will do harm and that the strongest stimuli always destroy. Classical medicine seems to have a preference for strong medication, the stronger and more concentrated the better, thereby often destroying the extremely sensitive natural symbiosis, the ecosystem of our brain and nerve centres. As long as modern medicine does not understand this, its remedies will always harm the patients in the long run. The only remedies I recommend in the case of too much stress are homoeopathic and other natural remedies.

Some people can cope much better with physical and mental stress than others; it depends on our personality, our way of life, our medical history and many other factors. Whenever there is stress we should try to get rid of it as soon as possible, and find a way of adjustment in order to lose our nervous tension.

WHAT STRESS MEANS TO BABIES AND SMALL CHILDREN

Some babies are quiet and seldom cry. Other babies cry very often indeed and once in a while even seem to be inconsolable. A baby is a very sensitive little creature and when its parents are under severe stress, it will react accordingly. A baby can also be stressed when it is dressed too warmly, when there is too much noise, when it feels pain and above all when its tummy hurts and its baby formula is wrong. A baby can become irritable, nervous, suffer from sleeplessness and even can become very angry when something is bothering it too much. Babies need lots of love and affection.

As you know already after reading the previous chapters, baby formulas and the nutrition of children from any age group are sometimes lacking in many of the most needed nutrients. Sweet foods are often low in vitamins and minerals, and high in saturated fats. Sugar becomes a serious problem when sweets, cakes and other snack food replaces more nutritious foods. Children need a balanced diet for normal growth and development.

Although we do not seem to realise it, in our industrial countries it is not easy to find a child that is really healthy. Most children, especially those living in towns, are often listless and tired. They lack vitamins, minerals and other nutrients needed to fight and prevent stress.

Small children who are still unable to express their stress in words will show it by their actions. They will suffer from anxiety and nightmares, become irritable, hyperactive, aggressive and afraid of sleeping alone; they may cower, run and bite, suffer from sleeping problems, or become accident-prone. Small children may even revert back to more immature behaviour, like sucking their thumbs, and fully toilet-trained children will suddenly start to wet their beds again. They may throw tantrums more frequently, or withdraw and become far too quiet.

The more severe the stress and the longer it lasts, the less control a child has over his or her reactions. The problem is that nowadays changes in our society and the lives of our children take place faster and faster, and the human organism cannot cope with so much stress. Parents should always try to prevent children being exposed to overwhelming stress, but this does not mean trying to keep them from experiencing normal, often healthy stressors. Children should learn that stress is a part of life and they should learn how to handle it. A sense of humour is extremely important. One should try to revert a negative into a positive stress.

ENDORPHINS

Endorphins are natural opiate-like chemicals made in the body, which enable it to relax, and give a feeling of well-being. Endorphins and other mood-enhancing neurochemicals are made from specific amino acids. Those of us who are deficient in these amino acids, and those who also lack essential vitamins, minerals and/or fats, suffer depression, low energy, cravings and anxiety.

When there are too few endorphins in the body of a child, the child becomes restless and unhappy much sooner than other children, and needs more care, cuddling and attention in order to feel a normal sense of happiness. It has been proved that children whose parents were drug addicts or alcoholics have a very low level of endorphins in their body. Children of addicts who do not become substance addicted themselves often suffer symptoms from a depleted biochemistry such as depression, exhaustion and mood swings

Modern life does not permit most parents to spend sufficient time with their children and instead of the mental support and understanding from their parents, these children will try to find other ways in order to calm down, when feeling lonely or unhappy.

When given a teaspoon of sugar in its formula, a small baby soon finds out that this sweet-tasting substance helps him to relax. We know now that sugar and several other foods and drinks trigger the release of endorphins. Most refined carbohydrates and stimulants, such as caffeine, and also many additives have the same effect. No wonder that we want to have more of these, because we like to feel happy and relaxed, instead of worried and unhappy.

Once, refined sweets and starches were the most popular drug foods. Now there are hundreds of comfort foods and drugs that have a far stronger effect. Whether it is alcohol, coffee, tea, sweets, cigarettes, sedatives, painkillers, cocaine and so on, all these addictive substances are means people use in order to feel better.

Realising how many food addicts, coffee addicts, sugar addicts, chocolate addicts, tobacco addicts and many other addicts there are in our modern society, we should not be amazed that the biochemical make-up of many of these people is not what it should be. Most people nowadays have a chronic lack of certain vitamins, minerals and other essential nutrients and the children who inherit their weakened constitution are the victims of the bad living and eating habits of their parents.

Many of us are bound to find relief where we can, in alcohol, cocaine, sugar, marijuana etc. Unfortunately, in addition to other side-effects, these drugs make the original deficiencies worse. Sugar and sugary drinks are the first substance that children become addicted to, but the problem is that sugar and all refined carbohydrates are not real food and do not contain the natural nutrients which the body needs in order to be and stay healthy. This is one of the main reasons why diabetes, now also found frequently in children, is one of the most feared diseases of our time.

CRAVINGS AND ADDICTION
One of the most important things you must understand about

addiction is that alcohol and addictive drugs are basically painkillers. They chemically kill physical or emotional pain and alter the mind's perception of reality. They make people numb. For drugs to be attractive to a person, there must first be some underlying unhappiness, sense of hopelessness or physical pain. Addictive substances not only let us forget our troubles, but also stimulate the part of our brain that is devoted to pleasure.

For example, somebody who has a personal problem may drink a few glasses too many. If this happens too often, biochemical changes take place in his body, whereby the body is depleted of some special nutrients, enzymes or hormones. After some weeks or months the same person may get into the habit of drinking more and more. However, now the craving for alcohol has little to do with the original reason for drinking. The more a person drinks, the greater becomes the lack of nutrients and at the same time the need to drink increases. Many people are caught up in a vicious circle, which lies at the bottom of many different kinds of addiction.

As soon as they feel some real or imagined stress, children can get into the habit of wanting a sweet or a soft drink. This habit becomes stronger and stronger, and because of the increasing chemical imbalance, often grows into an almost unbearable craving for sweets. This craving can be so bad that when I hear children yelling as if they are being murdered in the supermarket, I know, even from a distance, that they are trying to force their mothers to buy sweets or crisps for them.

The mothers of such children are usually overtired and as they do not want their children to yell in public, give in to their tantrums. Each time these children get the stimulant they desire their bodies are depleted of nutrients more and their addiction to non-food increases. As long as this goes on children cannot be healthy, but as a result of their addiction often develop enormous willpower, so that their parents feel helpless and may even become frightened of their own children.

At home, the children are the bosses and their wishes are catered to. Only a few people realise that these children are already devastated human beings, who need love and affection even more than other children of the same age. They become known as 'difficult to handle' and as they seem to reject personal contact they only receive a minimal portion of affection and care. Their own attitudes towards their parents and other members of the family prevent them from getting the very thing that they need most in life. Often their parents are unaware of their needs, and too damaged themselves to care for their children.

In ideal circumstances parents should give their children all the love and support they can during the first five or six years of their lives. After this time it should be easy for parents and their children to become good friends.

SCHOOLCHILDREN

When children start going to school, parents can relax, as part of their work will now be taken over by the teacher. However, a teacher has no time to concentrate on individual pupils and a child that at home was already a 'problem child' also becomes a problem in class, even for the most dedicated teacher.

We are living in a society that is very achievement-oriented. We bring up our kids to have high expectations and they will do anything in order to fit in, be admired and be part of the crowd. Most kids are not natural leaders and as a result they may feel nervous and bad about themselves. This often interferes with their learning abilities and although most of them are not at all stupid, they may lose their self-confidence and become depressed.

Sensitive children become emotionally harmed and often develop protective patterns to cover up for their imagined shortcomings. In the classroom they start cheating and lying in order to save themselves, because mistakes in the classroom are punished with public humiliation, reprimands and low marks. These are very powerful psychological weapons.

In the playground they follow the self-pronounced leaders, even if they do not really like them. In order to comply with classroom conditions children must give up their natural feelings of independence, dreams and feelings. Many children abandon their unique personality when they are in school. In order to survive, they must learn to act against themselves and not speak up on their own behalf. In this way they try to adjust to negative circumstances and adapt a second personality, a survival personality. Because of this, most children suffer from severe stress that can only be alleviated after school. Boys especially will start fighting and screaming, and get up to all kinds of mischief in order to get rid of their nervous tension.

Children need guidance and someone to hold on to; without it young children feel lost and afraid, and have no self-assurance. When it is missing at home, children have a tendency to follow the wrong kind of leader. At school many of these leaders are bullies who need to feel superior and try to force their ideas on the other children. They are the first to smoke, drink alcohol and take drugs, and humiliate other children who do not follow their example. Bad eating and living habits and the usual ill health, tiredness, hyperactivity, sleeping problems and general weakness do the rest.

CAFFEINE

Caffeine intake often begins early in life and the amount of caffeine consumed generally continues to increase throughout adolescence. Soft drinks are the main source of caffeine in most children's diet. It can be found in many foods, including chocolate and cocoa beverages, and is also an ingredient in many over-the-counter (OTC) medications. One dose may contain 200 mg of caffeine, as much as four or five cans of caffeinated fizzy drinks. Caffeine stimulates the nervous system and often causes nervousness, anxiety and disrupts sleep or restlessness. It is one of the first substances children can get addicted to.

By weight, children of one to five years of age consume the most caffeine. A three-year-old who drinks 8 ounces of caffeinated pop is getting as much caffeine as a 150-pound adult who drinks 1 litre.

Once children are hooked on sweets and/or caffeine, they give in to their addiction as soon as they feel a little nervous or restless. However, we should realise that soft drinks often take the place of nourishing food and rather than nourish, deplete the body of many valuable nutrients.

It is interesting to observe the incredible increase of caffeine-containing soft drinks in the last 100 years. The following example concerns Coca-Cola. In 1886 Dr John Pemberton invented Coca-Cola in Atlanta, Georgia, and in the same year the soft drink was sold to the public for the first time. Sales for that first year added up to a total of about 50 dollars.

By the late 1890s, Coca-Cola was one of America's most popular soda-fountain drinks and at the turn of the century the drink was sold across the United States and Canada. Until the 1960s, both small-town and big-city dwellers enjoyed these and other carbonated beverages at the local chemist or ice-cream saloon, where the soda fountain served as a meeting place for people of all ages. From this time on more and more people also bought soft drinks for consumption in their homes. In the last 30–40 years soft-drink sales have soared. Today, products of the Coca-Cola company are consumed at a rate of more than 1 billion drinks per day.

Since they came on the market, children have loved the soothing, relaxing and numbing effect of sugar and caffeine in soft drinks. But after getting used to these drinks, they soon realise that many other substances can also give them the same relaxed feeling, only more intensely. Soft-drink dependence seems to be the forerunner of alcohol, tobacco and drug dependence.

CHILDREN UNDER PRESSURE
Our children are caught up in a vicious circle from which many of them will never be able to escape. Children want to belong and are terribly afraid of being ostracised by the clan. Because of this it is very difficult to reach out and help them. Young children in particular can be put under pressure to take alcohol, or even drugs, by their friends. Although everyone has the right to say no, most children say yes because they are afraid of losing their popularity.

There is a common link to the way the brain responds to the sensuous aspects of sweets, soft drinks, alcohol and other stimulants. Each time that children are tempted to try out new stimulants, their dependency on such crutches increases.

These problems lie in nutritional and biochemical imbalances, rather than a lack of willpower or character. We have to look outside of psychiatry for solutions to the problem of addiction.

ALCOHOL
Many boys and girls of as young as 11 and 12 years old start experimenting with alcohol and surveys show that their most

popular drinks are beer, lager and cider, and sometimes spirits. Fizzy alcopops have become very popular and usually the alcohol content of these drinks is quite high.

Children drink mainly to alter their mood or cope with stress, because they want to feel happy and forget their problems; this is much easier when the brain is numbed. By drinking alcohol they also bond more with friends and the exploring of sexual relations becomes easier.

A related aspect is the partial merging of the alcohol and drug scenes in the context of youth culture, with alcohol being one of a range of psychoactive products now available on the recreational drug market.

HEAVY DRINKING AND ALCOHOL PROBLEMS

In Scotland more than half of 14-year-old schoolchildren reported having been drunk. Alder Hey hospital in Liverpool reported that children as young as eight were being admitted with acute alcoholic intoxication. In 1986, just 20 children were treated at Alder Hey for alcohol intoxication; by 1996 the figure had increased ten-fold to 200. This increase in cases was not restricted to Liverpool. Figures from accident and emergency units across the country suggest that around 50,000 teenagers are now being admitted with acute alcohol intoxication each year.

Alcohol-related problems include reduced performance at school, quarrels and arguments, sexual problems, fights, vandalism, driving accidents and many different health concerns. When drinking is combined with smoking, health risks are still greater.

Evidence shows that alcohol misuse while young is associated with heavy and problematic drinking in later life. There is also an association between alcohol, especially heavy drinking during teenage years, and the use of illegal drugs.

By and large, children follow their parents' example. Heavy-drinking parents tend to produce children who become heavy drinkers. Excessive alcohol consumption in adolescents may be related to low levels of parental support and control. A report from America found that young people are four times more likely to develop alcohol dependence than those who began drinking at the age of 21.

SMOKING

Children become aware of cigarettes from an early age. By the age of 11 one-third of children, and by 16 two-thirds, have experimented with smoking. In Great Britain about 450 children start smoking every day. In 1982, the first national survey of smoking among children found that 11 per cent of 11- to 16-year-olds were smoking regularly.

Children are three times as likely to smoke if both of their parents smoke and parents' approval or disapproval of the habit is also a significant factor. They are also influenced by their friends' and older siblings' smoking habits. Advertising reinforces the urge to smoke, creating the impression that smoking is a socially acceptable norm.

SMOKING AND CHILDREN'S HEALTH

The earlier children become regular smokers and persist in the habit as adults, the greater the risk of dying prematurely. A recent US study found that smoking during teenage years causes permanent genetic changes in the lungs and increases the risk of developing lung cancer later in life, even if the smoker subsequently stops.

Children are also more susceptible to the effects of passive smoking. In households where both parents smoke, the children are on average receiving a nicotine equivalent of smoking 80 cigarettes a year. Children of parents who smoke during the child's early life run a higher risk of cancer in adulthood and the larger the number of smokers in a household, the greater the cancer risk to non-smokers in the family. Several hundred people die every year from lung cancer caused by passive smoking – breathing other people's tobacco smoke. About half of all regular cigarette-smokers will eventually be killed by their habit.

Parents who smoke each year cause 8,000–26,000 new cases of childhood asthma in the US and make existing asthma worse in 20 per cent of the 2–5 million children who already have the disease. The saddest thing is that a recent survey reported that in 2000, 18 per cent of women continued to smoke during pregnancy in England.

ADDICTION

Children who experiment with cigarettes quickly become addicted to the nicotine in tobacco. Over half (58.5 per cent) of regular smokers aged between 11 and 15 years say that they would find it difficult to go without smoking for a week, while 72 per cent think they would find it difficult to give up altogether.

Every year, between 80,000 and 100,000 children become addicted to tobacco worldwide. Almost a quarter of Britain's 15-year-olds – both boys and girls – are regular smokers.

During periods of abstinence, young people have withdrawal symptoms similar to those experienced by adult smokers.

SMOKING PREVENTION

Since the 1970s, health education about the effects of smoking has been included in the curricula of most primary and secondary schools in Great Britain, but this does not seem to affect smoking rates.

Raising prices of cigarettes can deter children from smoking. A recent American study has shown that while price does not appear to affect initial experimentation with smoking, it is an important tool in reducing youth smoking once the habit has become established.

DRUGS

Whether it is sweets, soft drinks, coffee, tea, chocolate, sedatives, painkillers, alcohol, cigarettes, cocaine, heroine, crack, marijuana or other addictive substances, most people seem to need crutches in order to make their life bearable. These substances stimulate the 'reward' centre of the brain, and despite their varied nature, the pathways of the brain affected are extremely similar.

In primeval times the original cravings for sweets, starches and fats, as well as the chewing of certain relaxing herbs in times of danger, were needed for the survival of the human race. Now the very same cravings have become addictions for millions of human beings, especially young people, who seem to need stronger and stronger stimulants and tranquillisers in order to survive. However, many new substances threaten to overpower and kill us instead of giving relief. The long-term use of alcohol or drugs can lead to changes in the brain structure. Such adolescents live in a perpetual haze and most of the time do not realise what they are doing. Without doubt this has much to do with the constant growing crime rate.

Educational and health organisations have tried to halt this dangerous development, but most young people do not realise the danger and often couldn't care less. They do not worry about getting lung cancer when they are old, reasoning that 'We've all got to die of something.' Teenagers have a strong belief in their own immortality – 'It won't happen to me.' For young people it is hardly possible to estimate the personal risk.

State and privately funded schools alike are overrun by the drug problem. It is hardly ever possible to catch a drug supplier without a tip-off and most pupils are far too scared to tell for fear of violent retribution. Death threats are not uncommon.

British surveys suggest that 45 per cent of people aged 16–29 have used illegal drugs. It is estimated that 1.5 million ecstasy pills are taken every week in Britain. The Home Office believes that heroin addiction alone accounted for £1.3 billion property crimes in 1997. One in five of all people arrested are heroin addicts.

As a consequence of bad living and eating habits and the lack of much-needed nutrients, many grown-ups suffer from biochemical deficiencies that are later inherited by their children. Our children are a mirror image of our industrial world. While destroying our soil, our water and our air, we are also destroying the health of our children. Children who are addicted to tobacco, alcohol and drugs cannot possibly recover without help, but all our measures to change the prevailing tendency of self-destruction in our youth will be a waste of time, effort and money as long as we do not see the whole picture.

THE ORIGINS OF DESTRUCTIVE ADDICTIONS

It all starts in the cradle, or even before children are born. Addictive behaviour inherited from parents, sweets, soft drinks and junk food, and the resulting restlessness, hyperactivity or autistic behaviour, lie at the bottom of most of the increasing tendency for addiction.

From kindergarten on children can get into the quicksand of ever-escalating temptations and in order to get them out of the spiral of addiction, we must change our own attitudes in a very drastic manner. We all have a tendency to put the blame for the present sad situation on other people. We blame the cigarette and alcohol industries, publicity, television and drug cartels. Of course all of those do a lot of harm, nobody who loves their children will deny this, but we should keep in mind that all business is always a question of supply and demand; whenever products are sold successfully, it means there is a heavy demand for them.

Why is there such a heavy demand for these health-endangering products? Why do our children need stimulants and tranquillisers? There are many different reasons, but most are closely related to the fact that many of our children are not really happy. They have a feeling of uselessness and of being lost. They do not understand their role; they see the futility of our modern way of life. Many parents cannot give them the stamina they need in order to withstand temptation and on the contrary often show them a bad example.

> The youth is directly reflecting the crisis on Earth. The water is poisoned and no longer safe to drink without filters. Our soil is exhausted through erosion, top-soil depletion, and billions of tons of pesticides. Our soil is void of life and vitality, needed to grow food that can nourish our children's bodies. While polluting our air, water and soil, we are polluting our children.
>
> (Earth in a crisis)

Somewhere along the road real values have been lost and in order to help our children, we should find them again.

We are weak. We have lost our courage and willpower. We are watching our children drowning, but we ourselves have never learnt to swim and we do not know how to save them. Hundreds of thousands of us join political protest marches: we want a different government, we want better leaders, who will fight alcohol, tobacco and drugs and make life worthwhile and safe again. But what honest and honourable man wants to be a leader in our time, a leader of people who are weak and do not even have the courage to change their own lives? People who do not protest when their fields and farmlands, their water and the air they breathe are being poisoned for the sake of money and so-called progress. People who accept that once-wholesome food, that once served to build a healthy and courageous people, is being changed into artificial products that would be inedible without many thousands of additives, colourings and taste-makers. People who accept that their children have become alcoholics and drug addicts, without trying to give up their own bad habits. Most people have lost belief in themselves, they are weak, even weaker then their own children, who are the real victims.

Of course there are still are some people who try to fight, to do the right things, but they are only a small minority and most people nowadays are of the opinion that it is better to do nothing at all, rather than take a risk. Millions of us go to church every Sunday, but during the week we forget the promises we made and do nothing, while watching our children drown.

When I was young, we ate simple and wholesome food and we still knew how to be happy and play simple games. Most modern children do not know how to play simple games any more. They are used to videogames, where winning, shooting, killing and the subjection of others is of the greatest importance. Modern children need these games, however, in order to know how to defend themselves in real life.

For our young children we buy noisy toys that can harm their hearing beyond repair. When these children grow up they need even more noise in order to get a feeling of being unimpeachable and strong. The weaker their personality and the more hopeless and downtrodden teenagers feel, the more noise they will make to regain some of their lost self-assurance.

Many children, especially those living in towns, do not know the wonderful feelings of happiness and peace one can find in natural surroundings; they do not know any more how to daydream while listening to the song of birds or watching the clouds. They do not know that all living things, plants, animals and human beings, have their own special place in the centre of things. Nature is the best teacher. As soon as children have the opportunity to observe nature by themselves they will be able to understand it, and by and by they will lose their feelings of loneliness and incompetence.

Everything living in the world – plants, animals, tiny insects and human beings – has its own very special assignment. Every human being, every child, has a unique personality and special talents that nobody else has. All life is interlocked, and all forms of life need one another. Everyone is responsible for the health and welfare of all children. The only way to get out of the spiral of addiction, towards a free and happy life, is to start, not tomorrow but today, to change our own lives and save the children that still can be saved.

Most children don't know the joy of living any more. Start by giving your children more care, more fun and above all more love and understanding. Do things together with your children – hiking and camping, or sailing and rowing. Let them know that you need them and show them nature, birds and flowers. Explain to them that all human beings are responsible for their own lives. Teach them the value of healthy food and a healthy lifestyle, and never say 'no' without explaining 'why'. Shake yourself up – drink less alcohol, coffee and soft drinks, eat fewer sweets and less junk food, stop smoking, and try to show your children in everything you do that you are fighting your own bad habits, because happiness is worth fighting for. Your head will become clear again and life will be much happier. Your example is the most important thing for your children. They will be proud of you and will learn to be proud of themselves.

I once read: 'The greatest phase in man's advancement is that in which he passes from subconscious to conscious control of his own mind and body'; this saying has become my favourite quotation. No human is born to be a slave, either of other people, or of their own weaknesses. All human beings have the inborn material for further development and greatness and should learn to use what is given to them, so that they can be proud and happy.

The first thing young people must learn is to have the courage to stand up and resist the influence of others in their life. They should be honest with themselves and live according to their own beliefs of what is right and wrong for them. I would love to tell all young people: 'Jump from the bandwagon and start the adventure of living your own life. Escape when there still is time and you still have the willpower to do it. It will be not always be easy, you will have to learn much and work hard until you are really independent, but you can do it. Anything is better than being the chattel and slave of some self-appointed leader and his or her dependant and feeble-minded groupy. Take the road of real happiness, from the slavery of addiction towards freedom.'

INDEX

acne 100

AD/HD (Attention Deficit Hyperactive Disorder) and ADD (Attention Deficit Disorder) 16, 50, 51, 55–6, 57, 58, 59, 97, 100, 105; homoeopathic treatments 131–7; psychiatric counselling for 125–30; drug treatment for 122–5; and violence 153

addiction 162–73; and children 161–2, 163, 165–9; illegal drugs 169–70

adipic acid 114

adrenaline 158–9

aggression 46–9, 54, 106, 110–11, 135

alcohol 150, 162–3, 166–8

alkaline metabolism 88

allergic responses 69, 80–5, 143 154; and behavioural problems 81, 82–3; causes 81–2; common problems 8; and everyday substances 82; testing for 84–5; understanding of 82–3;

aluminium 97, 99

Alzheimer's disease 99

amalgam 25, 98–9

analgesics 102

animal testing 64–5

antibiotics 60, 63

antioxidants 114

Argenticum nitricum 134, 135–6

Arsenicum 134, 135

ascorbic acid 151

aspirin 102, 113, 114

asthma 52, 81, 82, 104, 113, 133, 136

Atrazine 60

autism 16, 56–7, 59, 81, 93, 99, 100, 104, 110, 111

baby food 30, 31, 37, 43–5

baby milk see formula

bed-wetting 54

behavioural disorders, spectrum of 15–17, 30–1, 46–9, 50 see also AD/HD; hyperactivity

biochemical disorders 52, 141–4

blood sugar levels 26, 73, 75–9, 154

boron 106

breakfast 76, 77, 78

breast milk 33, 80, 99

breast-feeding 29–30, 33–42

Breggin, Peter B. 142

cadmium 60, 97, 100, 153

caffeine 68–9, 81, 165–6

Calcarea phosphoricum 134, 136

calcium 69, 76, 87–8, 104–5

cereal 81, 84

Chamomilla 134–5

chemical products 118–21

chocolate 81

cigarettes, see nicotine; smoking

Cina 134, 135

colostrum 33

conception, healthy 18–23
constipation 52, 54, 156
coordination, lack of 55
copper 21–3, 97, 99–100, 106, 107, 153
cosmetics 103, 104, 115
cows' milk 30, 35–6, 39, 47–8, 80–1, 84, 87, 106, *see also* formula
criminal behaviour 149–54

detoxifying 155–7
Dexedrine 124
diabetes 71, 75–6, 93
diarrhoea 52, 54, 81, 114
dysgraphia 50, 51
dyslexia 50, 51

E numbers, details of 112–17
ear infections 51, 54, 133
ear, development of 27–8, 108–11
eczema 52, 81, 104, 105
eggs 81, 84, 104
endorphins 161–2
enemas 156–7
eyesight problems 56

fatigue 54
fatty acids 103, 107
Feingold Diet 105, 116
folic acids 106, 107, 151
food additives 61, 63–6, 69, 89–93, 113–17; colourings 112–13; consumption rates of 92; indirect 94–5; to avoid 117
food intolerances 85
food legislation 91
foods/ingredients to avoid 115–117
formula (baby milk) 30, 32, 35, 36, 80–1, 87, 99
Freudian theory 127
fungicides 98

gene disorders 128
genetically modified foods 60

hair tests 21, 106, 107
hearing: in babies and children 108–11
herb teas 74, 78, 107; varieties 138–40

homoeopathic remedies 131–7, 157
hormones 63
Hyoscyamos niger 134, 135
hyperactivity 15–17,66, 69, 73, 77–8, 81, 90, 92, 100, 106, 109; symptoms of 53–7; homoeopathic treatment for 131–7; drug treatment for 122–5; and psychiatric counselling 126–30
hyperglycaemia/hypoglycaemia, *see* blood sugar levels

impotence 20
infertility 19–23
insulin 72–3, 75
intestinal flora 57
intestines, cleansing 155–7
iron 106, 107
irritable bowel 105

junk food/fast food 52, 55, 61, 64, 144; and violence 151–4; weaning children off 78–9, 116

Kalibromatum 134,136
kidney damage 98, 100, 104

lead 25, 60, 97–8, 153
learning disabilities 50–2, 55, 100
light, health effects of 145–8
lipstick 103
low self esteem 56, 164–5, 171
Lycopodium 134, 136

magnesium 106
MBD (minimal brain dysfunction) 16
medicine, modern 118–21
Medorrhinum 134,136
Mendelsohn, Dr Robert 122
mercury 21, 25, 59, 60, 97, 98–9
metal pollutants 96–101
'miasma' 132
migraine 105, 114, 148
milk, *see* cows' milk
monosodium glutamate 81, 114, 115
morning sickness 26

nicotine 24–5, 168–9
nitrates/nitrites 114
noise level standards 108–9

noise pollution 28, 108–11, 132–3, 172; and toys 108, 172
nutrients, lack of essential 106–7, 141–4, 150–4, 161

obesity 68, 93; in babies 36
oil, processing of 83–4, 152
orthomolecular medicine 141–4
Ott, John 146

packaging 63, 84, 94, 103, 114
Pasteur, Louis 118
Pauling, Linus 141
peer pressure 166, 173
Peoline 124
pesticides 60, 63, 98
Pfeiffer, Dr Carl 32, 49, 152
pharmaceutical companies 118–20
phosphorus 61, 73, 79, 86–8
pineal gland 147
potassium 106
pregnancy; and noise 109; and nutrition 24–9
preservatives, see food additives
processed/refined foods 63–4, 73, 104 see also junk food
protaglandins (PGs) 103
psychiatric counselling 126–30

Ritalin 16, 122–5

salads 78
salicylates 102–5, 115
school snacks 78
selenium 106
Selye, Hans 158, 159
skin problems 52, 81, 104, 105, 113, 136
smoking 24–5,168–9; passive 168
sodium 100, 106
sodium caseinate 114, 116

soft drinks 67–70, 165–6
soil pollutants 60–1, 84, 86–7
sorbates 113
soya milk 36
sperm quality 20
stevia 74, 78
Stramonium 134, 135
stress 158–61; in babies and small children 160–1
sugar 62, 67, 71–9, 162; addiction to 162, 163, 165; and allergies 81; in soft drinks 67–8; and violence 152–4 see also blood sugar levels
sulphites 113

Tarantula hispanica 134, 135
Thiordazine 124
thyroid dysfunction 112
Tomatis, Dr Alfred 27–8, 111
tooth decay 68, 93
traffic 111
tranquillisers 120–1
triclic drugs 124

vaccination 58–60
vanadium, 100–101
vegetable milk 36–7
Veratrum album 134, 136
vitamin B3 151
vitamin B6 106, 107
vitamin B12 106, 107
vitamin D 76, 87, 146

Walsh, Dr William 152–3
water contamination 61
Westernisation 93
wet-nursing 38–42

zinc 22–3, 100, 106, 107, 153